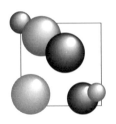

*Plasma and Recombinant
Blood Products in
Medical Therapy*

Molecular Medical Science Series

Series Editors

Keith James, University of Edinburgh Medical School, UK

Alan Morris, University of Warwick, UK

Forthcoming Titles in the Series

Introduction to the Molecular Genetics of Cancer *edited by* R. Vile

Molecular Biology of Immunosuppression *edited by* M.R. Walker and R. Rapley

Molecular Genetics of Human Inherited Disease *edited by* D.J. Shaw

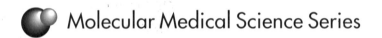 Molecular Medical Science Series

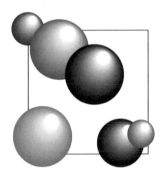 *Plasma and Recombinant Blood Products in Medical Therapy*

Edited by
CHRISTOPHER V. PROWSE
Director, National Science Laboratory,
Scottish Blood Transfusion Service, Edinburgh, UK

JOHN WILEY & SONS
Chichester · New York · Brisbane · Toronto · Singapore

Published 1992 by John Wiley & Sons Ltd
        Baffins Lane, Chichester
        West Sussex PO19 1UD, England

Other Wiley Editorial Offices

John Wiley & Sons, Inc., 605 Third Avenue,
New York, NY 10158–0012, USA

Jacaranda Wiley Ltd, G.P.O. Box 859, Brisbane,
Queensland 4001, Australia

John Wiley & Sons (Canada) Ltd, 22 Worcester Road,
Rexdale, Ontario M9W 1L1, Canada

John Wiley & Sons (SEA) Pte Ltd, 37 Jalan Pemimpin #05–04,
Block B, Union Industrial Building, Singapore 2057

Library of Congress Cataloging-in-Publication Data

Plasma and recombinant blood products in medical therapy / edited by
    Christopher V. Prowse.
        p.   cm. — (Molecular medical science series)
    Includes bibliographical references and index.
    ISBN 0 471 93200 0
    1. Recombinant blood proteins—Therapeutic use.   2. Blood
products.   I. Prowse. Christopher V.   II. Series.
    [DNLM: 1. Blood Transfusion.   2. Plasma.   WB 356 P7125]
    RM171.4.P53 1992
    615'.39—dc20
    DNLM/DLC
    for Library of Congress   91–43676
                                                              CIP

British Library Cataloguing in Publication Data

A catalogue record for this book is
available from the British Library

ISBN 0 471 93200 0

Typeset by Inforum Typesetting, Portsmouth
Printed in Great Britain by Biddles Ltd, Guildford

Contents

Contributors

Nuala A. Booth BSc, PhD
Lecturer, Department of Biochemistry, Marischal College, University of Aberdeen, Aberdeen

Jan E. Boyd BSc, PhD
Research Associate, Department of Surgery, University of Edinburgh Medical School, Edinburgh

Thierry Burnouf BSc, PhD
Director of Fractionation, Centre Régional de Transfusion Sanguine, Lille, France

Peter R. Foster BSc, PhD
Director of Research and Development, Protein Fractionation Centre, Scottish National Blood Transfusion Service, Edinburgh

H. Anne Leaver BSc, PhD
Senior Scientist, Edinburgh and South East Scotland Blood Transfusion Centre, Edinburgh

Moira C. McCann BSc, PhD
Head of Immunology and Cell Biology, National Science Laboratory, Scottish National Blood Transfusion Service, Edinburgh

Shirley L. McDonald BSc
Research Associate, National Science Laboratory, Scottish National Blood Transfusion Service, Edinburgh

Ron V. McIntosh BSc, PhD
Principal Scientist, Protein Fractionation Centre, Scottish National Blood Transfusion Service, Edinburgh

Ian R. MacGregor BSc, PhD
Head of Biochemical Studies, National Science Laboratory, Scottish National Blood Transfusion Service, Edinburgh

Alex J. MacLeod BSc, PhD
Principal Scientist, Protein Fractionation Centre, Scottish National Blood Transfusion Service, Edinburgh

Sarah M. Middleton BSc, PhD
Manager of Product Development and Regulatory Affairs, Delta Biotechnology, Castle Court, Nottingham

Steve Moore BSc, PhD
Head of Molecular Biology, National Science Laboratory, Scottish National Blood Transfusion Service, Edinburgh

William G. Murphy MD, MRCP, MRCPathol
Senior Lecturer in Transfusion Medicine, Edinburgh and South-East Scotland Blood Transfusion Service, Edinburgh

Chris V. Prowse BSc, DPhil, MRCPathol
Director, National Science Laboratory, Scottish National Blood Transfusion Service, Edinburgh

Robert R.C. Stewart BSc, PhD
Clinical Trials Manager, Scottish National Blood Transfusion Service, Edinburgh

Peng Lee Yap BSc, MB ChB, PhD, MRCPathol
Consultant, Edinburgh and South-East Scotland Blood Transfusion Centre, Edinburgh

To Ruth, Ben, James and Jane in view of the time I have devoted to this
book, rather than to them

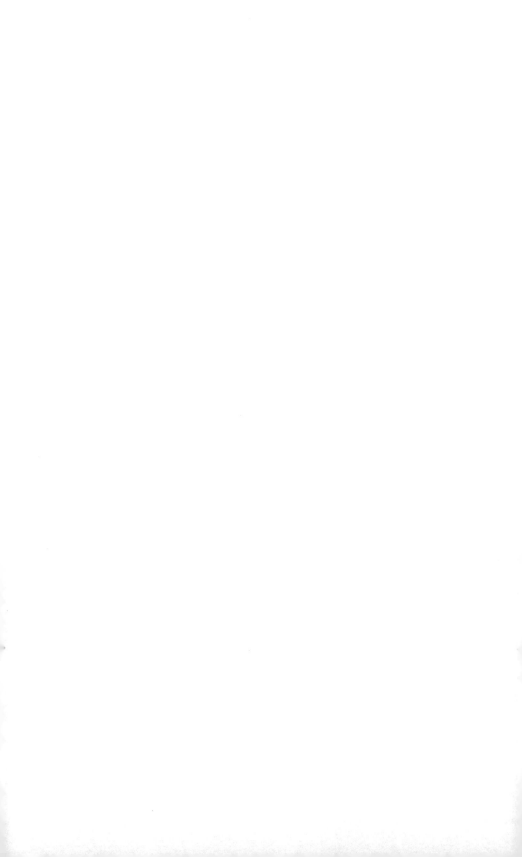

Acknowledgements

In preparing this book, the editor has been helped by many colleagues from within the Scottish National Blood Transfusion Service, as well as friends from elsewhere. I would like to thank them all for their time and help and point out that any views expressed by them or myself in this book are personal ones, rather than those of the organizations for which they work. Finally, I would like to express my gratitude to Dr Keith James and Dr Brian McClelland for their continued advice and encouragement.

1 Introduction

C.V. PROWSE

The idea behind this book came from the realization that molecular biology is perceived as coming of age. Many people are now discussing the use of recombinant products for therapy of patients. In some cases this offers the only route of providing the product. In other cases there is the promise of replacing a conventional product.

For those working in the field, many of whom started their careers before the potential impact of molecular biology was realized, the term 'blood products' has a fairly restricted meaning. It is usually interpreted as those therapeutic products that are prepared from (human) blood. In general this is the meaning that has been assumed for this book. Molecular biology has enabled us to widen this definition to include a range of materials that are present in blood but have not been conventionally prepared, for therapeutic use, from that source. Some examples of this are discussed in the sections on fibrinolysis, cytokines and growth factors at the end of this book.

The intention behind this book is to provide a primer, for those interested in the use of therapeutic blood products, of how we have arrived at the current state of the art and what advantages or disadvantages molecular biology may offer. It is not intended to provide an extensive review of the fields involved, but suggestions for further reading are included at the end of each chapter.

In developing any therapeutic product, the prime concerns have to be whether it will be useful, safe and effective in the patient. The editor has therefore chosen to start this book by considering what factors are involved in assessing products for patient use. This is followed, in Chapter 3, with a description of the conventional approach to fractionation of human plasma into therapeutic products – providing coagulation factors, immunoglobulin and albumin.

The next two chapters review the newer technology, covering the general approaches as to how to use molecular biology to prepare therapeutic products, and recently developed methods of purifying products from plasma or molecular biological sources. Finally, recent developments in specific areas are considered.

Plasma and Recombinant Blood Products in Medical Therapy
Edited by C.V. Prowse.   Published 1992 by John Wiley & Sons Ltd

Table 1.1 Some important dates in the development of blood products and recombinant technology*

Year	Blood products	Year	Recombinant technology
1945	Description of plasma fractionation by E. Cohn's group	1953	Watson and Crick model DNA structure
		1954	Salk polio vaccine from cell culture
1950s	Early coagulation factor concentrates	By 1960s	Description of bacteriophage and plasmid structures
Early 1960s	Poole's description of cryoprecipitate	1968	Description of restriction enzymes (Smith, Nathans and Arber)
Late 1960s	Routine therapeutic use of coagulation concentrates		
1970s	Development of intravenous immunoglobulin and intermediate purity coagulation products	1974	Kohler and Milstein describe monoclonal antibodies
		1975	Sanger describes method for sequencing nucleic acids
		1977	Genentech founded
1983	Recognition of viral agent causing AIDS	1981	Cloning of human albumin
Late 1980s	Development of viral inactivation technology and high purity coagulation factor products	1982	Therapeutic use of recombinant insulin
		1984	Cloning of Factor VIII
		1986	Therapeutic use recombinant t-PA
		1987	Clinical trials of recombinant Factor VIII

See Appendix 2 for a list of cloned blood protein genes.

To provide a background to the current situation, Table 1.1 provides a few crucial dates in the development of blood products and recombinant technology. It includes the establishment of the company Genentech as it is largely through such specialist companies that recombinant therapeutic products have been developed as a real possibility.

During the 1980s genes for many of the proteins in blood were cloned (see Appendix 2). The potential thus exists to develop any of these as recombinant therapeutic products.

Apart from safety and efficacy, the factors considered in determining whether a product is better prepared from blood (or plasma) or by molecular biology largely relate to cost. To develop a recombinant therapeutic takes tens of years and tens, if not hundreds, of millions of pounds and, unlike the multiple useful products present in plasma, each project will probably only yield one product. The questions to ask may include:

- *How much is needed?*
  It is obviously easier to provide a few grams of Factor VIII than tons of albumin.
- *Is there an alternative source?*
  Products such as Factor VIII and albumin are already made from plasma. Others, such as cytokines or plasminogen activator, cannot be made from this feedstock while some, such as α_1-protease inhibitor, may not be available in sufficient amounts from plasma.
- *How much will it cost to produce?*
  For a recombinant product the answer will indubitably be – a lot! Cost may differ by orders of magnitude if the product can be prepared in microorganisms rather than mammalian cell culture, or if the product is a relatively small simple molecule such as insulin, rather than a large complicated one, like Factor VIII.
- *What will it cost to purify?*
  Unlike plasma products, recombinant ones are usually made from sources that contain non-human proteins and nucleic acids derived from culture media or cells. There are extensive guidelines on such matters (see Appendix 5). These include demonstrating the absence of infective agents, such as viruses, and the need to show minimal levels of contaminating protein and nucleic acid in the final product. If one considers levels of 10 µg protein or 10 pg of nucleic acid as the maximum level of contamination acceptable per dose, then a 1 mg dose of Factor VIII requires a protein purity of 99%. This may sound difficult but pales into insignificance when compared to the corresponding 99.9999% purity for a 10 g dose of albumin. The costs of consistently achieving and demonstrating such purification may well exceed the costs of production.

Given the restrictions imposed by the answers to the above questions, it is doubtful if more than two or three manufacturers will find it worthwhile to prepare any one viable recombinant product. Against this background, it is hoped that this book will be of interest to those new to, or already working in, the fields of blood transfusion, biological pharmaceuticals and haematology, as an update of the newer developments and options for blood product provision.

2 Clinical Aspects

R.R.C. STEWART and W.G. MURPHY

THE USE OF BLOOD PRODUCTS IN CLINICAL MEDICINE

Proteins extracted from human blood or plasma, or such proteins manufactured by other processes, have two main functions in clinical medicine.

1. To replace the lack of these substances in individuals, for example the use of Factor VIII:C (FVIII:C) in patients with haemophilia A.
2. To supplement the natural production of such substances to induce a therapeutic effect in patients suffering from a disease not caused by, or associated with, a lack of such substances. An example of this is the use of high-dose intravenous immunoglobulins in idiopathic thrombocytopenic purpura.

The major products in terms of the blood products industry are FVIII:C, albumin and intravenous immunoglobulin. Other products are coagulation factors other than FVIII:C and immunoglobulins other than intravenous IgG.

FACTOR VIII:C AND HAEMOPHILIA A

FVIII:C is used exclusively for the treatment of haemophilia A. Congenital haemophilia A is caused by diminished or abnormal production of FVIII:C. The disease is inherited as an X-linked recessive disorder. It is expressed in affected males and carried by the affected females, of whom only a rare individual will have clinical disease. The genetic defect may consist of deletional or missense mutations. Most cases will be born into a previously affected family; however the FVIII:C gene has a high mutation rate, and about 20% of congenital cases arise from *de novo* mutations. Haemophilia A is the commonest of the hereditary coagulation disorders, with an incidence of about 7 per 100000 males at birth.

Occasionally, haemophilia A can be caused by autoantibodies to FVIII:C arising in adult life. In these cases the disease can be associated with other immune disorders such as systemic lupus erythematosus, or with drugs such as α-methyldopa.

Plasma and Recombinant Blood Products in Medical Therapy
Edited by C.V. Prowse.   Published 1992 by John Wiley & Sons Ltd

Patients with haemophilia A do not tend to bleed from small superficial wounds; bleeding is typically internal, in weight-bearing joints and in traumatized muscles. In addition, haemophiliacs are prone to serious intercranial bleeding from minor head trauma, and this is the principal cause of haemorrhagic death.

The absence of FVIII:C predisposes to abnormal bleeding by interference with physiological coagulation mechanisms.

THE FORMATION OF THE BLOOD CLOT

Disruption of the endothelial lining of the blood vessel precipitates a series of complex events that leads in turn to (1) formation of a platelet plug, (2) formation of a fibrin clot on the platelet plug and (3) endothelial cell regrowth and dissolution of the clot.

Once the platelet plug is formed, a cascade of serine proteases is activated on the phospholipid surface of the plug. These proteases are derived from inactive proenzymes in the plasma, or in the platelet granules. The localized activity of enzymes is increased exponentially by feedback loops and requires the presence of non-enzymic co-factors (see Chapter 6).

Deficiency or impaired function of any of the many factors involved in the formation of the platelet plug or of the fibrin clot results in a bleeding disorder. FVIII:C is an important non-enzymic co-factor in the enzyme cascade. Deficiencies of other components of the enzymic pathways lead to very similar diseases. Such deficiencies have also been described for the protease precursors Factor VII, Factor IX, Factor X, Factor XI and prothrombin and for the co-factor Factor V. In general, the severity of these diseases does not differ from that of haemophilia A. They are less important to the blood product industry mainly because their prevalence is less.

THE REQUIREMENT FOR FACTOR VIII:C

FVIII:C concentrate is given to patients with haemophilia A either to treat an established bleeding episode, or to prevent bleeding in certain settings. No source of FVIII:C other than concentrate is currently recommended.

The amount of FVIII:C given for a bleeding episode usually varies with the site and severity of the bleed. It is usual to attempt to raise the plasma FVIII:C concentration above a specific therapeutic level, and repeated doses are given to maintain the desired level as necessary, or until the bleeding stops. The amount of FVIII:C infused to prevent bleeding also varies with the circumstances.

Some patients with severe haemophilia (< 20%) develop IgG antibodies to infused FVIII:C. These patients have an impaired haemostatic response to treatment with FVIII:C. The severity of this impairment varies from patient to patient. In some patients, no therapeutic responses can be achieved with very high doses of FVIII:C. In others, a useful response is achieved with infusions of about 200 U/kg body weight followed by infusion of 1000 U/h.

SOURCE OF THERAPEUTIC FACTOR VIII:C – CLINICAL CONSIDERATIONS

FVIII:C for clinical use in haemophilia can be derived from human plasma by fractionation, yielding low-, intermediate-, or high-purity concentrates, or can be derived from recombinant gene technology. Purity of FVIII:C preparations is expressed as units of activity per milligram of total protein. Levels > 100 U/mg can be achieved by fractionation techniques mainly involving the use of either ion-exchange chromatography or immuno-absorption chromatography. Much lower levels (< 1–10 U/mg) are the rule for other fractionation methods and for recombinant preparations. The low levels in recombinant FVIII:C concentrates are due to the necessity of adding albumin to the final preparation for FVIII:C stability. All preparations are sterilized to inactivate the human immune deficiency virus and viruses causing hepatitis B and hepatitis C. At least one known virus, parvovirus B19, may survive current sterilization methods. This virus can cause a transient bone-marrow suppression and can lead to clinical disease in patients with severe congenital anaemia, such as sickle-cell anaemia or thalassaemia major, or in patients with other intercurrent disorders of red-cell production or survival. Clinical disease due to B19 has not been observed in haemophiliacs, although almost all patients have antibodies to the virus, as do many otherwise healthy people. However, the resistance of this virus to current sterilization techniques indicates that a potential for viral transmission remains.

Reduction in contaminating proteins in FVIII:C preparations is probably, but not necessarily, a good thing. There is no proven advantage, and this will be difficult to resolve unequivocally. Theoretical advantages include diminished likelihood of contamination with unknown viruses, and diminished immune dysfunction due to infusions of large amounts of non-FVIII proteins. For example, it has been shown that plasma-derived FVIII:C concentrates inhibit lymphocyte proliferation, interleukin-2 expression, and natural killer cell activity, but the clinical relevance of these findings is unknown.

One theoretical drawback to the use of high-purity FVIII:C concentrates is that the hypothetical reduction in immune suppression could lead to an increase in the incidence of patients developing antibodies to FVIII:C; this has not been demonstrated.

Those who treat patients with haemophilia A are in agreement that in the present state of knowledge, the purer the product used the better, provided that supply is not compromised; any FVIII:C preparation that does not transmit HIV is better than none at all. It is to be expected that, failing unforeseen clinical problems with recombinant FVIII:C, this product will eventually be a major source of FVIII:C in those countries that are able to pay for it.

FACTOR IX

Inherited deficiency of Factor IX (FIX) causes haemophilia B, a disease that is clinically indistinguishable from haemophilia A. The principles of treating or preventing the bleeding in haemophilia B are the same as those of haemophilia A. FIX is infused in the form of plasma-derived concentrates to achieve and maintain the desired levels.

Use of concentrates of FIX has the same problems as those of FVIII, such as viral transmission and immune dysfunction. In addition they have been implicated in the unwanted production of a hypercoagulable state in some recipients. This has been associated with the occurrence of thromboembolic disease (deep venous thrombosis and pulmonary emboli, as well as with arterial thrombosis). This complication arises particularly in patients undergoing major operations, such as joint-replacement surgery in the lower limbs.

Contaminating coagulant factors (other than FIX) are thought to be the major contributors to this adverse effect. Trace amounts of serine proteases in active forms, such as Factors IIa, VIIa and Xa may be the causative factors. FIX concentrates in current use are all plasma derived. No recombinant protein has been produced in therapeutically useful amounts.

Most of the plasma-derived concentrates contain significant amounts of the other coagulant and anti-coagulant vitamin K-dependent serine proteases: Factors II and X, and Proteins C and S. Some concentrates also contain Factor VII.

As discussed in relation to FVIII concentrates, a high-purity FIX concentrate is clinically desirable, probably more so in the case of FIX (because of the reduced risk of thrombogenicity). Such concentrates, with specific activity of at least 10 U/mg total protein, have recently become available.

OTHER CLINICAL USES OF FACTOR IX CONCENTRATES

FIX concentrates are currently used in two other settings. Clinical indications for FIX therapy other than haemophilia B are:

(1) disease states associated with multiple clotting factor deficiencies (e.g. warfarin therapy, liver disease or gastrointestinal disease); and
(2) bleeding in patients with haemophilia A and antibodies to FVIII:C.

Bleeding in association with multiple clotting factor deficiencies

Although FIX-containing concentrates are not the first line of management in these patients, they are sometimes necessary to provide adequate control of bleeding. Factor VII-deficient concentrates require the addition of Factor VII. High-purity FIX concentrates will be even less appropriate for these patients. Clinical demand will persist for mixed concentrates of Factors II, IX and X, although an alternate therapeutic route may be to use recombinant Factor VIIa.

Bleeding in patients with haemophilia A with inhibitors to FVIII:C

Inhibitory antibodies to FVIII:C arise in up to 20% of patients with congenital haemophilia A. As discussed above, some of these patients will respond to large doses of FVIII:C, others will not. Several options are available for treating these patients: none is universally successful. Products used in the treatment of haemophilia A with inhibitors are:

- Large doses of FVIII:C concentrate
- FIX concentrate
- Activated prothrombin complex
- Porcine FVIII:C
- Recombinant activated Factor VII

In controlled trials, FIX concentrates produce a haemostatic response in 50% of episodes treated. Activated concentrates produce a similar response. The mechanism of action is uncertain, and may be related to the presence of some activated Factor VII (Factor VIIa) in the preparations. Factor VIIa reduces the need for FVIII:C in the generation of thrombin. This mechanism underlies the use of recombinant Factor VIIa discussed below.

FACTOR VII

RECOMBINANT ACTIVATED FACTOR VII

Recombinant Factor VIIa (rFVIIa) has been introduced as an agent to bypass the need for FVIII:C to achieve *in vivo* haemostasis in patients with inhibitory antibodies to FVIII:C. Although possibly not as effective in clinical use as FVIII:C when adequate levels of FVIII:C can be achieved, rFVIIa represents a significant advance in managing haemophilia A in patients with inhibitors. It is also effective in haemophilia B with inhibitors, and it is worth remembering that it is acceptable as a treatment for clotting factor deficiencies in those patients whose religious beliefs preclude the use of blood products. This product may also prove to be useful in place of combined concentrates of Factors II, VII, IX and X in bleeding associated with oral anticoagulants, malabsorption and liver diseases.

FACTOR VII DEFICIENCY

Congenital FVII deficiency is a rare autosomally inherited disorder. The symptoms include bleeding from mucous membranes, and easy bruising.

FVII deficiency arises in some disease states such as liver disease, warfarin therapy and malabsorption.

In congenital cases FVII concentrates prepared by plasma fractionation are the treatment of choice. Good response can be obtained by infusions of plasma alone, but the use of sterilized factor concentrate is safer than un-sterilized plasma and avoids possible problems due to volume overloading.

Therapy with factor concentrates is occasionally necessary in acquired factor deficiency due to liver or gastrointestinal disease, or to warfarin therapy. FVII concentrate may be added to FVII-deficient concentrates of Factors II, IX and X in these settings.

VON WILLEBRAND FACTOR

Preparations of von Willebrand factor (vWf) for infusion are necessary for the treatment of some patients with von Willebrand's disease (vWD).

vWf is a large multi-functional protein synthesized in endothelial cells and megakaryocytes. It is essential for platelet adhesion to sites of endo-thelial injury, and as a carrier protein for FVIII:C *in vivo*. It is also involved in platelet-to-platelet aggregation. The protein naturally occurs as a large poly-mer. In its absence, patients have a bleeding disorder characterized by easy bruising, mucosal bleeding, menorrhagia and internal (especially muscle and joint) bleeding.

The clinical picture is highly variable between, and within, the individ-ual patients, and severe forms of the disease are present only in a minority of cases. There is a variety of sub-types of the disease, depending on whether the underlying biochemical defect is one of reduced synthesis, impaired formation or stabilization of polymers, synthesis of dysfunction-al forms of the molecule, or most commonly, impaired release from sites of storage.

In the majority of patients, those with some synthesis of the normal multimeric forms of the molecule, infusions of vWf-containing prepara-tions is rarely – if ever – required. However, severely affected patients do require replacement therapy with vWf for treatment and prevention of bleeding episodes. Some, though not all, FVIII:C concentrates contain use-ful amounts of functional vWf for therapeutic use in patients. As discussed in respect to FVIII:C earlier, a purified or recombinant vWf preparation would have several advantages over the currently available products. Re-combinant vWf has been expressed in several cell types, and in multimeric forms closely resembling those in normal plasma. However the use of such vWf in patients with vWD would require the addition of FVIII:C to the preparation, since the FVIII:C levels are also low in severe vWD. Following vWf infusion, endogenous FVIII:C levels rise. However for the treatment of bleeding episodes, this rise may be too slow for adequate haemostasis, so that some FVIII:C is also required in therapeutic preparations of purified vWf.

Recombinant fragments of vWf have also been expressed. These fragments may contain only one of the functional sites of the molecule, for example the binding site for platelet membrane adhesion. Such fragments can inhibit platelet function *in vitro* and in animal models, and may be exploited in future as an injectible anti-platelet agent.

ALBUMIN

The current use of albumin preparations worldwide is about 100 tonnes per year. The level of use per number of inhabitants varies greatly between different countries in the developed world. The variation would seem to have more to do with availability and cost than with medical need.

Albumin is available in preparations of 4.5–5% (5% albumin, plasma protein solution, plasma protein fraction) and of 20%. It is prepared from pooled human plasma, and after 40 years of clinical use has an enviable safety record. Correctly manufactured, there have been no reports of transmission of known viruses. Previously contaminating prekallikrein activity was implicated in causing hypotension during rapid infusion of albumin solutions. This risk has now largely been eliminated. Inherent in the nature of the product is the risk of causing fluid overload in the recipient, leading to cardiac failure. This is particularly the case with 20% albumin.

The 4.5–5% albumin is indicated in several clinical settings:

- Plasma volume replacement in shock syndromes
- Replacement of protein in burned patients
- Replacement fluid in therapeutic plasma exchange

Within each of these settings the exact requirements for albumin have not been completely established, and in many instances substitution of albumin with other colloid solutions such as gelatin, or with crystalloids, such as saline, is not associated with unfavourable clinical effects.

The 20% albumin is indicated for the treatment of diuretic-resistant oedema in hypoproteinaemic patients, and for use in exchange transfusions in neonates.

Patients with excessive protein loss through the kidney, gastrointestinal tract, or skin, or with diminished protein production in the liver, are prone to develop oedema, with contraction of the intravascular fluid compartment, and compensatory salt retention. Such oedema can be resistant to diuretic therapy, but may respond to infusions of 20% albumin at doses of 20–40 g/day.

In the absence of any serious problems with currently available plasma derived albumin, the pressure to produce a recombinant product is less than for other plasma derived products, apart from normal human IgG, and the task facing potential manufacturers of recombinant albumin for therapeutic use is a daunting one. However, a recombinant albumin preparation might be desirable as a stabilizing additive to recombinant replacement proteins such as FVIII:C, as the risk of life-long exposure to plasma-derived albumin is not known. It is possible, for example, that the use of human albumin over long periods may induce immune dysfunction in recipients, due to contamination with other plasma-derived proteins. Therefore, recombinant FVIII:C with *plasma derived* albumin added as a stabilizer, may be less attractive than recombinant FVIII:C with recombinant albumin stabilization.

IMMUNOGLOBULIN PREPARATIONS

Both specific and non-specific immunoglobulin preparations are used in clinical practice. Specific immunoglobulin (IgG) preparations are available for treatment or prevention of a number clinical diseases. These preparations are derived either from fractionation of pooled selected human plasma, or are produced by biotechnology methods.

Non-specific, or more properly 'multi-specific', immunoglobulin preparations are also widely used, and for a growing number of clinical indications. These products are prepared by fractionation of non-selected human plasma. This product of the plasma fractionation industry is at present the least amenable to replacement by engineered non-plasma derived products. This is mainly because, for many uses, the important constituents of the preparations are not identified, and it is possible that a mixture of a large range of antibody specificities, including anti-idiotype specificities, may be needed for the therapeutic effect. In addition, for use in preventing infections in immune deficiency states, the intravenous IgG preparation needs to contain antibodies to many pathological organisms to be clinically useful.

Non-specific preparations of human IgG in current use include normal human immunoglobulin for intramuscular injection and IgG for intravenous infusion.

Normal human immunoglobulin for intramuscular injection is now mainly used for hepatitis A prophylaxis, and may also be useful in preventing rubella infection after exposure.

INTRAVENOUS IgG

Preparations of IgG from pooled human plasma suitable for intravenous injection (IVIgG) were originally introduced as replacement therapy for patients with hypogammaglobulinaemia, both congenital and acquired. It is an effective replacement therapy. Some instances of hepatitis (non-A,non-B) have been reported, and minor side effects such as fever and tachycardia have been observed occasionally.

A major use for IVIgG preparations has been in the treatment of some autoimmune disorders, the most notable of these being auto-immune thrombocytopenic purpura (ITP). In this disorder, the patients develop an autoantibody to platelet membrane structures. In children the condition commonly arises after an upper respiratory tract infection; in adults such an association is unusual. The antibody-coated platelets are rapidly removed by the effector cells of the reticuloendothelial system, particularly by the splenic macrophages. The resultant thrombocytopenia leads to a tendency to bleed.

Over two-thirds of patients achieve remission of disease following infusion of 1–2 g IVIgG/kg body weight (i.e. 4–8 times the dose used for replacement therapy in hypogammaglobulinaemic patients). In most patients, the effect is only short-lived, but in some it is sustained.

The ability to introduce brief remissions is valuable in preparing patients for surgery or for obstetric labour. It can also be exploited as a long-term strategy for patients with recurrent severe bleeding.

As well as autoimmune thrombocytopenic purpura, several other auto-immune and alloimmune disorders have proved responsive to high-dose IVIgG. The exact mechanism of action of IVIgG in these settings awaits elucidation, before the potential for reproducing the effect by biotechnological methods can be evaluated.

SPECIFIC IgG PREPARATIONS

Examples of specific antibodies derived from human plasma from donors with high levels of specific antibodies are shown in Table 2.1.

Table 2.1 Specific antibodies from donor human plasma

Anti-Rhesus D	Prevention of haemolytic disease of the newborn Prevention of Rhesus sensitization in other settings
Anti-hepatitis B	For prevention of infection following exposure to hepatitis B infection; e.g. in babies born to infected mothers
Anti-varicella zoster	For prevention of varicella (chicken pox) infection in patients who have been in contact with an infected person, and who have impaired immune defences (e.g. newborns, patients receiving myelosuppressive chemotherapy)
Anti-cytomegalovirus	Treatment of cytomegalovirus infection in immune-suppressed individuals, e.g. following organ transplantation
Anti-tetanus	Treatment or prevention of infection following exposure
Anti-rabies	Prevention of infection following exposure

NON-PLASMA DERIVED IMMUNOGLOBULIN PREPARATIONS

Bioengineered immunoglobulin preparations have a vast potential for the treatment of a large number of clinical conditions. This is an area of intense development (see Chapter 8). Preparations in current use, or in advanced stages of development, include: (i) monoclonal antibodies to T-cell subsets for the treatment of organ graft rejection *in vivo*, and *ex vivo* for T-cell depletion of bone marrow harvested for allogeneic transplant; (ii) human monoclonal antibodies for the treatment of bacterial endotoxaemia; and (iii) anti-drug monoclonal antibodies for the removal of toxic levels of digoxin. In clinical use, monoclonal antibodies have been associated with reactions ranging from fever to circulatory collapse. Transmission of viral diseases by such preparations has not been reported.

PHARMACEUTICAL DEVELOPMENT OF BLOOD PRODUCTS FOR CLINICAL USE

Plasma protein products are pharmaceuticals and as such are covered by the local pharmaceutical regulations. In the UK these regulations are detailed in the Medicines Act 1968 and the guidance Medicines Act Leaflets (MALs) published by the Department of Health and latterly by the Medicines Control Agency. A plasma protein product for routine use should have a product licence (marketing authorization). The use of products on a 'Named Patient Basis', i.e. for specific patients without such a licence, should be avoided where possible.

The stages in assessing a pharmaceutical product in man are conventionally split into four clinical phases:

Phase one: Short-term pharmacokinetic and pharmacodynamic studies to determine the safe dose in humans. For most products these studies are normally performed on healthy (male) volunteers. However as all plasma products have an inherent risk of transmission of blood-borne viruses, it is not considered acceptable to use healthy volunteers.

Phase two: Small studies in which patients (persons likely to gain benefit from the administration of the product) are exposed to the product for the first time.

Phase three: Larger studies which build on and expand the knowledge gained from the earlier studies. These studies provide the bulk of the safety and efficacy data which have to be supplied for a product licence (marketing authorization) application.

Phase four: The transition from Phase three to Phase four is marked by the granting of a product licence. Studies performed in Phase four usually are either to gain further information on the safety of the product (post-marketing surveillance) or to look at other indications for the product which are not covered by the established product licence.

According to the regulatory procedures in the UK, it is normal practice to perform initial human studies with a new chemical entity drug on healthy volunteers. These can be performed without the need to submit the study for approval by, nor even to register it with, the Medicines Control Agency. The prudent researcher, however, will seek the approval of a local ethics committee. However, plasma protein products should not normally be given to healthy volunteers. While all efforts may be made to eliminate known viruses, no absolute guarantee can be given that a product derived from human blood (or any other source that is potentially infectable by viruses) is entirely free from the risk of transmission of infectious agents.

When patients are to be exposed to a new drug for the first time, either a Clinical Trial Certificate (CTC) or a Clinical Trial Exemption (CTX) should be applied for. A CTC application requires that full details of the following be supplied:

- Chemistry (of the active substances)
- Pharmacy (of the formulation)
- Pharmacology
- Toxicology
- Carcinogenicity
- Volunteer studies

The assessment of a CTC application normally will take 9–12 months and once granted is valid for two years.

A CTX application requires the same data as the CTC application but only in summary form. Either a company medical adviser or a consultant to the company signs a statement that they have reviewed the data and that the summary supplied is a true representation of the whole data, and that in their opinion the product is safe to administer to humans. The Medicines Control Agency has 35 days to assess a CTX application (which may exceptionally be extended by a further 28 days) and, once granted, a CTX is valid for three years.

However, as has been noted earlier, this process cannot be strictly adhered to for plasma products, as volunteer studies are not appropriate. Thus, it is necessary to apply for a CTX (CTC) for a plasma product before it is given to any humans and only persons likely to gain benefit from the product (by definition, patients) should be exposed to it. Thus, with a plasma product, studies such as pharmacokinetic studies should be performed in patients under a CTX or CTC.

Before a sufficiently large group of patients in a pharmacokinetic study are exposed to the new product, a very small number of patients should receive it in hospital or a specialized clinical research establishment with resuscitation facilities on hand, lest there be some unforeseen and severe reaction to its administration.

The objective of a pharmacokinetic study with a plasma protein product is to demonstrate that the processing which the product has undergone has not altered the molecule in such a way as to change its *in vivo* half-life or in any other way to materially alter its inherent properties. This is an ideal which has had to be compromised at times, for example when reduction/ sulphonation of immunoglobulin was necessary to remove the anti-complementary activity prior to its use intravenously.

Once it has been shown that the product has an acceptable recovery and half-life, the product can enter the next stage of its clinical development, at which time it becomes necessary to demonstrate that the product is effective. This may be relatively easy for some products and will require a relatively small study, e.g. the demonstration that FVIII stops bleeding, or it may require a larger more complex study as has been the case with demonstrating that intravenous immunoglobulins reduce the incidence of infections in hypogammaglobulinaemic patients.

Assuming that the plasma product has been shown to have an acceptable recovery and half-life and to be effective, it then is necessary to perform carefully monitored clinical trials which should be designed to assist in the identification of the unusual adverse event. It should be noted however that any truly idiosyncratic reaction is unlikely to occur until the product is in routine use, as such reactions occur with a low frequency in the population at risk.

The obvious objective is to produce a safe product. However, it is impossible to define safety. Rather an acceptable risk rate should be set *a priori* and a clinical trial designed to test this rate. In most cases, the medical researcher should seek the advice of a statistician. A particularly interesting case is where the rate should be very low and in fact no events are seen during the study. How sure can we be that the true rate is low? This depends on the number of patients at risk, as the upper 95% confidence limit of the estimate is given by the so-called rule of three:

$$\text{Upper 95\% confidence limit} = \frac{3}{\text{Number at risk}}$$

A study which follows, for example, 500 haemophiliacs treated with a FVIII product and shows no development of antibodies to hepatitis C would have an upper 95% confidence limit for the true rate of 1 in every 166, while in a similar study which monitored 60 patients with the same result would have an upper 95% confidence limit of 1 in 20.

Once the data from these studies are accumulated, the application for a product licence can proceed. The Regulatory Authorities will require that you demonstrate that the product is efficacious, that it is safe and that it is of pharmaceutical grade. If these three major criteria can be satisfied, then a licence will be granted, although it is very common for the Authorities to request further information during their consideration of an application.

Plasma-derived proteinaceous products should be treated in a manner analogous to a new chemical entity developed by a pharmaceutical company. Ideally, it should not be supplied for routine use until it is granted a product licence and throughout its development it should be subject to the same constraints and level of monitoring as any new pharmaceutical product.

FURTHER READING

Aronson, D.L. and Menache, D. (1987) Prevention of infectious disease transmission by blood and blood products. *Progress in Hematology*, **15**, 221–241.

Berkman, S.A., Lee, M.L. and Gale, R.P. (1990) Clinical uses of intravenous immuno-globulins. *Annals of Internal Medicine*, **112**, 278–292.

Dollery, C.T. and McClelland, D.B.L. (1991) Dextran and albumin. In: *Therapeutic Drugs, A Clinical Pharmacopoeia* (Ed. C.T. Dollery). Churchill-Livingstone, Edinburgh.

Medico-Pharmaceutical Forum. (1987) Report of the Working Party on Clinical Trials of the Medico-Pharmaceutical Forum. Royal Society of Medicine Services, London.

Yap, P.L. and Williams, P.E. (1990) Novel intravenous immunoglobulins and their applications. *Baillière's Clinical Haematology*, **3**, 423–449.

3 The Principal Elements of Plasma Product Manufacture

P.R. FOSTER and R.V. McINTOSH

INTRODUCTION

Comparatively recent developments in molecular biology and immunology have increased general awareness in the potential use of proteins as macro-molecular drugs. However, proteinaceous products have been established in clinical use for many years and are an essential feature of modern medicine. In contrast to biosynthetic (e.g. recombinant materials), established pharmaceutical proteins are derived from blood plasma supplied by human donors. The frac-tionation of human plasma into different constituents has enabled a range of high-quality clinical products to be manufactured worldwide on an industrial scale, the principal products being albumin solutions (for volume replacement and the treatment of shock), immunoglobulin preparations (for the prevention and treatment of infectious diseases and immune disorders) and coagulation factor concentrates (for the prevention and treatment of bleeding disorders).

About 15 million litres of plasma are processed annually worldwide and it is important to emphasize that plasma fractionation is a process industry manufacturing complex pharmaceutical products, rather than a laboratory operation. In this chapter we will first describe factors which constitute the framework which determines the nature of the manufacturing operation and how it can be carried out. This will be followed by a description of the principal unit process operations used by the industry to manufacture plasma products for clinical use. Detailed preparative methods are not presented as these are already well described in references listed at the end of the chapter for further reading.

THE MANUFACTURING FRAMEWORK

REGULATION AND CONTROL

The preparation of plasma products for clinical use is a pharmaceutical manufacturing operation and as such is governed by the same regulatory

Plasma and Recombinant Blood Products in Medical Therapy
Edited by C.V. Prowse.   Published 1992 by John Wiley & Sons Ltd

considerations that apply to the wider pharmaceutical industry.

In the UK, Manufacturing and Product Licences must be obtained from the Medicines Control Agency, while product specifications are described in the European Pharmacopoeia and are monitored and controlled by the National Institute for Biological Standards and Control. Similar arrangements exist in other countries and, although there may be some variations in standards, there is an increasing trend towards harmonization.

GOOD MANUFACTURING PRACTICE

A central feature of licensing is a requirement to comply with a set of standards known as Good Manufacturing Practice (GMP). These standards encompass the design of the manufacturing facility and its organization and operation and are intended to ensure that a high quality of manufacturing is achieved reliably.

The manufacturing premises

Clinical products must be sterile and free from pyrogenic contaminants. To achieve this, buildings and equipment must be appropriately constructed and maintained in a hygienic manner and sterile conditions must be available for the aseptic dispensing of products into their final containers. The flow of materials must also be designed to move logically from receipt of raw materials to product dispatch without crossing, so that any mix-up can be avoided. The movement of personnel must also be defined and controlled appropriately.

Documentation

A major feature of GMP is the need to have detailed, up-to-date, written descriptions of all tasks and procedures involved in the manufacturing operation. Such documents are known as Standard Operating Procedures (SOPs). It is also necessary to record methods used and parameters obtained at the time of manufacture in a standard descriptive document known as the Product Specification Batch Record (PSBR). Analytical measurements are recorded in an associated standard document known as the Quality Control Batch Record (QCBR).

Further areas which require documentation include:

- cleaning of facilities and equipment
- calibration and maintenance of instruments and equipment
- specification, purchase and testing of components and raw materials
- validation and control of manufacturing processes

- specification of intermediate and final products
- definition of systems for the storage and retrieval of documents, raw materials, intermediate products and final products

The purpose of such documentation is to provide a system of control, to instruct personnel in the procedures concerned, to ensure that these procedures are followed correctly and to provide a complete history of each batch of product.

Personnel

The people employed must be suitably qualified and trained for the tasks to be undertaken. Staff are grouped into different departments so that their primary functions and responsibilities can be clearly defined and appreciated. These normally include Production, Engineering Maintenance, Quality Control, Quality Assurance/Regulatory Affairs, Research & Development and Administration. To comply with GMP, it is essential that Quality Control should be independent from the Production management to avoid any potential conflict of interest when, for example, a batch of product is rejected.

MANUFACTURING OBJECTIVES

Plasma fractionation utilizes a valuable and limited human resource to manufacture life-saving products and its objectives must respect both the blood donor and the product recipients. This dual perspective enables a number of clear objectives to be identified, against which processing methods can be designed or selected.

Clinical safety

The manufactured product should be free from constituents which may be harmful to the recipient. These may have been present in the donor plasma (e.g. viruses) or introduced (e.g. bacterial pyrogens, toxic reagents) or generated (e.g. vasoactive substances, thrombogenic substances) during processing. Bacterial contamination must be minimized by carrying out processes using equipment and facilities of sanitary design. Chemicals introduced during processing may never be fully removed, and for this reason it is preferable where possible to avoid the use of substances which may be potentially toxic. In some instances, substances which may be responsible for adverse reactions are not known and in these circumstances it is not possible to guarantee that a product will be free from such effects no matter how pure it may be.

Product efficacy

The products must be presented with the desired component in a stable biologically active form and at the appropriate concentration for the intended clinical application. This may be difficult where the desired component is unstable or where the effective component is not known.

Production capacity

The process methods and technologies must be capable of operating at a capacity that will meet the anticipated product demand. This is particularly important for those manufacturers who aim to satisfy the needs of a defined population from its own blood-donor resource (e.g. national self-sufficiency).

Manufacturing economy

The costs of manufacture will normally be met by the community (either directly or indirectly) and by the blood donor who provides the process feedstock. Therefore it is incumbent on manufacturers to employ efficient and cost-effective processes and to avoid the use of unnecessarily complex (usually low yielding) or expensive procedures.

Industrial suitability

All process operations should be suitable for routine practice in a pharmaceutical manufacturing environment. As well as meeting the objectives outlined above, a process should be capable of being validated and controlled and should be easy to operate reproducibly and to integrate with adjacent manufacturing activities.

PROCESS INTEGRATION

Plasma fractionation involves the preparation of a range of different products from a common feedstock. A large number of manufacturing steps may be required (Figure 3.1) and each of these must be selected and designed to meet both organizational and process needs.

Organizational needs

The process routes to particular products are illustrated schematically in Figure 3.1. In its simplest form, the route to any product can be sub-divided into two stages. The first of these is the mainstream process (the solid line in Figure 3.1) where processing (for example, from 0 to d) ideally should not be

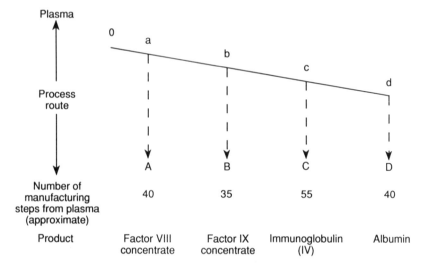

Fig. 3.1. Process integration: points at which off-line processing (- - - - - -) interacts with mainstream processing (————)

interrupted. The end result of the mainstream process is a number of inter-mediate products (i.e. at points a, b, c, d) which are further processed (i.e. to points A, B, C and D) to obtain the various products in their final form. This latter stage of processing (dashed lines in Figure 3.1) is carried out away from the mainstream process and can be regarded as an off-line operation. Ideally, off-line processing should be independent of the mainstream process, otherwise all products may be constrained (e.g. in terms of plant output) by the weakest step in any of the off-line processes. Similarly, a breakdown at any step would put all processes out of action. The ability to separate the organization of mainstream and off-line processing maximizes both capacity and operational flexibility and enables much of the manufacturing operation to continue in the event of an isolated breakdown of equipment or facilities. To achieve this, it is necessary to be able to hold intermediate products (e.g. at points a, b, c and d) for further processing at a later date. This can currently be done at points a, c and d by freezing the respective precipitates, e.g. cryoprecipitate, Fraction I + II + III and Fraction IV4 + V (Figure 3.2).

Process needs

Each step in a process fulfills a particular function and, as process yield normally decreases with increasing complexity, it is important that the number of functions is minimized and that they are carried out in the order in which they are most effective or efficient. Where possible, multiple functions should be combined into a single step. Generally it is helpful if process

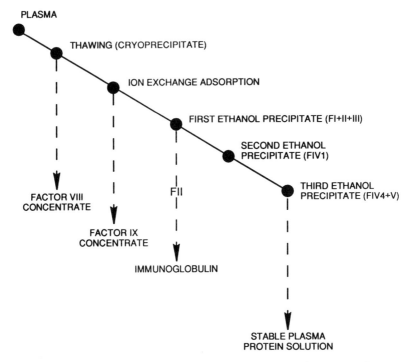

Fig. 3.2. Process scheme for the fractionation of plasma at the Protein Fractionation Centre (SNBTS). Stable plasma solution is a form of albumin

volumes can be reduced at an early stage with some degree of purification, as this reduces the quantity of material to be processed making less robust procedures (e.g. chromatography) easier to accommodate.

A process design must also achieve the requisite product specification and yield without introducing changes into shared process sections that adversely effect other products. For example, an apparently minor change in section 0–a (Figure 3.1) to increase the yield of coagulation Factor VIII could result in a profound change to the quality of the coagulation Factor IX concentrate being produced via route 0–a–b–B.

Process change

The design of changes to improve an existing process (e.g. to increase yield) or to introduce a new process (e.g. to obtain a new product) must accommodate both the organizational and process needs described above and an appreciation of these must be incorporated into process research and development from the beginning. The detailed implications of these points tend to be specific to each manufacturer's operation, and consequently it is

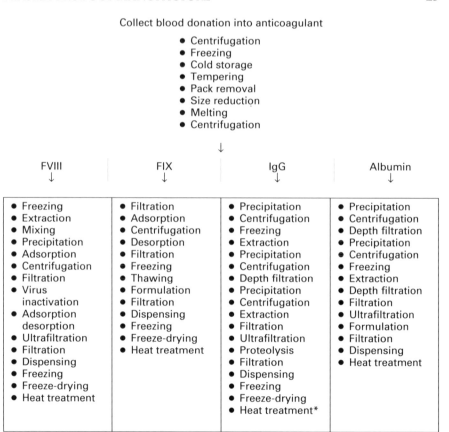

Collect blood donation into anticoagulant

- Centrifugation
- Freezing
- Cold storage
- Tempering
- Pack removal
- Size reduction
- Melting
- Centrifugation

↓

FVIII ↓	FIX ↓	IgG ↓	Albumin ↓
• Freezing • Extraction • Mixing • Precipitation • Adsorption • Centrifugation • Filtration • Virus inactivation • Adsorption desorption • Ultrafiltration • Filtration • Dispensing • Freezing • Freeze-drying • Heat treatment	• Filtration • Adsorption • Centrifugation • Desorption • Filtration • Freezing • Thawing • Formulation • Filtration • Dispensing • Freezing • Freeze-drying • Heat treatment	• Precipitation • Centrifugation • Freezing • Extraction • Precipitation • Centrifugation • Depth filtration • Precipitation • Centrifugation • Extraction • Filtration • Ultrafiltration • Proteolysis • Filtration • Dispensing • Freezing • Freeze-drying • Heat treatment*	• Precipitation • Centrifugation • Depth filtration • Precipitation • Centrifugation • Freezing • Extraction • Depth filtration • Filtration • Ultrafiltration • Formulation • Filtration • Dispensing • Heat treatment

* Operations under development at the Protein Fractionation Centre (SNBTS).

Fig. 3.3. Process operations used in the manufacture of the principal plasma derivatives prepared at the Protein Fractionation Centre (SNBTS)

often necessary for process advances to be selected and tailored by manufacturers to meet their individual needs.

Process unit operations

The overall process is made up of a large number of individual steps. The
major steps for each of the principle product routes are shown in Figure 3.3.
This rather complex picture can be simplified by combining the different
product routes into a generalized grouping of common process steps or unit
operations (Table 3.1). These steps and the principles on which they are
based will be described in the remainder of this chapter.

Table 3.1 Summary of unit process operations used in the manufacture of plasma products at the Protein Fractionation Centre (SNBTS)

Feedstock preparation	Blood donation
	Removal of cells
	Freezing of plasma
	Tempering of frozen plasma
	Pack removal
	Size reduction of frozen block
	Melting of frozen plasma
Protein separation	Fractional precipitation
	Fractional extraction
	Solid–liquid separation
	Adsorption/desorption
Storage of intermediate fractions	Freezing/thawing (liquids)
	Freezing/extraction (solids)
	Freeze drying
Product finishing	Adsorption (depth filtration)
	Ultrafiltration
	Selective proteolysis
	Membrane filtration
	Dispensing
	Freeze-drying
	Heat treatment

FEEDSTOCK PREPARATION

DONATION

Plasma for fractionation is provided by human donors in two ways – by whole-blood donation or by plasmapheresis. In the case of whole blood, the cellular components are separated from the plasma some time after donation whereas during plasmapheresis the separated erythrocytes are returned to the donor by intravenous infusion. This means that donations by plasmapheresis can be larger and more frequent than those given as a whole blood. Furthermore, because delays in processing can have an adverse effect on plasma quality, plasmapheresis plasma is generally considered to give a higher quality feedstock for fractionation.

ANTICOAGULATION

Sufficient anticoagulant is required during blood donation to prevent clotting of plasma and so allow its separation from the other components of whole blood. Sodium citrate has a long established use in plasma collection and fractionation as an anticoagulant. The use of citrate, however, also has an adverse effect on plasma quality in the chelation by citrate groups of Ca^{2+}

which are essential in maintaining the normal structure of Factor VIII. The stability of Factor VIII activity in plasma can be improved by using heparin as an anticoagulant and so avoiding the chelating effects of citrate and maintaining normal physiological levels of ionized calcium. Alternatively a mixture of Ca^{2+} and heparin has been added to citrated plasma immediately after harvesting to improve Factor VIII stability. There is also growing evidence that simply reducing the concentration of citrate in standard citrate–phosphate–dextrose–adenine (CPD-A1) anticoagulant to half its normal level significantly improves Factor VIII stability while maintaining effective levels of anticoagulation.

Any benefits in Factor VIII stability from changes in anticoagulant formulation which might improve the feedstock quality must be recoverable in the manufacturing processes used to prepare Factor VIII concentrates. Furthermore, any formulation changes must not interfere with the fractionation of other products from plasma, especially Factor IX concentrates which require adequate anticoagulation to prevent activation leading to thrombogenic components contaminating the final product. For these reasons, changes to anticoagulation must be carefully validated in the full-scale plasma fractionation process before being implemented in feedstock collection.

FREEZING AND THAWING

Plasma recovered from whole-blood donations or donated by plasmapheresis is stored frozen for later processing. Therefore, freezing and thawing of plasma are critical operations in industrial-scale fractionation. The aims are to preserve the important activities contained in the plasma and to recover these activities as efficiently as possible for further processing. These operations are of particular importance in the preparation of Factor VIII concentrates because virtually all methods of Factor VIII production begin with the extraction of Factor VIII activity from a cryoprecipitate formed during the freeze–thaw process.

Within the overall freeze–thaw process, four stages can be identified. These are:

(1) freezing (to less than –27°C)
(2) cold storage (at less than –27°C)
(3) the first stage of thawing involving the 'tempering' or 'conditioning' of the plasma (–10°C)
(4) the second stage of thawing where the plasma is melted into a liquid state (0°C to +2°C)

The use of appropriate end-point temperatures, determined by the freezing characteristics of plasma, and controlled rates of temperature change throughout the freeze–thaw process are essential to obtaining high-quality plasma and cryoprecipitate for further processing.

PACK REMOVAL

At some time during, or prior to, the processing of the frozen plasma to a liquid feedstock for mainstream fractionation, the plasma must be removed from its container. Since the frozen donations will range from <200 g to 500 g in weight and the throughput of a plasma fractionation plant can be measured in hundreds of tons, this is a major task in feedstock preparation. One approach is to carry out the whole thawing process (including melting the plasma) in the individual containers. However, this is clearly a labour-intensive method and dealing with large numbers of small units does not lend itself to the good temperature control throughout a batch, essential to the freeze–thaw process. One method of removing the plasma bags (or 'packs' as they are commonly known) is by immersion in liquid nitrogen causing the plastic to shatter. The frozen pellets of plasma can then be picked out from the freeze-fractured plastic and returned to temporary cold storage or continue into the thawing process.

It is also possible to remove the plastic pack during thawing since at the warmer temperature used for plasma conditioning (–10°C), the plastic is pliable enough and has lost sufficient of its adherence to the plasma to be stripped from it. In fact, warming of the plasma prior to melting was originally introduced to enable the plastic bag to be removed. This is currently achieved by either cutting the end from the bag or by slicing the donation in half (e.g. by using a toothless hygienic bandsaw).

OPPORTUNITIES FOR FURTHER DEVELOPMENT

There are many areas in which the quality of plasma as a feedstock for fractionation could be improved. In the formulation of anticoagulants, for example, despite demonstrations by several methods that Factor VIII stability can be improved in plasma by maintaining normal physiological levels of calcium, donations are still collected in a citrate concentration far in excess of that required for adequate anticoagulation chelating, the Ca^{2+} essential in maintaining Factor VIII activity.

Although the formation of a cryoprecipitate is a key step in plasma fractionation the mechanism of cryoprecipitation and its relationship to the freezing characteristics of plasma are still poorly understood.

Most of the methods used in the plasma fractionation industry for coping with a large volume of feedstock packaged in small units are manual and labour-intensive. The introduction of reliable automated pack removal systems compatible with the range of packs in use is long overdue.

PROTEIN SEPARATION

PRECIPITATION

Background

The dominant protein-separation method in plasma fractionation is precipitation, whereby proteins are separated according to their solubility differences. Solubility behaviour describes a unique property of a protein which is derived from its amino acid structure. The solubility of proteins is also a function of their environment; consequently a large number of parameters determine the actual solubility of an individual protein (Table 3.2). Some of these parameters are specific to each protein and cannot be changed except by chemical or biochemical modification of the native molecule. Other parameters can be changed relatively easily and their variation can be used to cause a selected protein or group of proteins to leave the solution phase, a process commonly known as 'precipitation'.

The use of high ionic strength to precipitate proteins (i.e. salting-out) was first recorded by Denis in 1859, with the importance of H^+ concentration subsequently being recognized by Sørenson, leading him to develop the concept of pH in 1917. By 1900, Osborne and Harris were using metal ions to precipitate proteins, while in 1908 Mellanby reported the precipitation of serum proteins by the addition of ethanol. These early practitioners had manipulated individual parameters (e.g. ionic strength), but to advance the method, a more comprehensive approach was required which would enable multiple parameters to be exploited simultaneously in a complementary manner. It was a student of Osborne and Harris, Edwin Cohn who in 1925 proposed a generalized empirical relationship to describe protein salting-out. This encompassed pH, temperature and

Table 3.2 Parameters which determine the solubility of proteins

Fixed	Variable	
Protein	Protein	Environment
Molecular size	Charge	pH
Molecular conformation	Ion binding	Dielectric constant
Amino acid composition		Ionic strength
Amino acid sequence		Temperature
Polar/non-polar residues		Solute:solvent ratio
chemical nature		Specific ion effects
ratio		
distribution		
Number of ionizable		
residues		
Dissociation constants		

individual protein characteristics as well as ionic strength and, known as the Cohn equation, remains in use today.

By 1940, Cohn and co-workers had utilized simultaneously five of the six variable parameters available (Table 3.3) to separate human plasma proteins into the major clinically important fractions. The preparation of a human albumin solution for volume replacement provided the impetus for the programme; however, methods were also obtained for the preparation of a range of other products including immunoglobulins, fibrinogen and antihaemophilic factor (Factor VIII). Albumin, prepared for clinical trial by Cohn's Method 6 at the laboratories of Harvard Medical School, was first used in 1941 for the treatment of casualties at the US Naval base at Pearl Harbor. The product was so successful that an immediate decision was taken by the USA authorities to establish full-scale manufacture using the facilities of pharmaceutical companies. Within 18 months, significant levels of production were being achieved on seven manufacturing sites. As a consequence of this wartime project, Cohn's Methods 6 and 9 (used for off-line immunoglobulin processing), or variants of them, became the central protein separation methods for the manufacture of plasma derivatives and remain so today.

Table 3.3 Principles of cold ethanol (Cohn) precipitation

pH	Protein solubility is usually at a minimum near its isoelectric point. Therefore pH is adjusted to the isoelectric point of the protein(s) to be precipitated but avoiding extremes of pH. Conditions intermediate between the isoelectric point of proteins present should be avoided to prevent the formation of insoluble protein complexes
Dielectric constant	Electrostatic forces involved in molecular interaction increase as the solution dielectric constant decreases. The dielectric constant is reduced by the addition of ethanol resulting in a reduction in overall protein solubility
Ionic strength	Solutions are held at low ionic strength so that small variations can be used to increase the solubility of specific proteins to promote separation. Such salting-in effects are enhanced at low dielectric constant (i.e. in the presence of ethanol)
Temperature	Protein solubility normally decreases with reducing temperature. Low temperatures are required to obtain complete precipitation but overshoot may result in precipitation of unwanted protein or freezing of the solution. The temperature must not exceed 0°C if denaturation is to be avoided and is preferably held well below 0°C
Protein concentration	Protein stability is normally reduced at low protein concentration. Hence dilution of the protein solution is avoided as much as possible

Process technology

Processing at the pilot plant of Harvard Medical School was carried out on 30-litre batches of plasma and the rapid scale-up of the method suggests that precipitation procedures are simple and straightforward. Although precipitation is well suited to large-scale operation, a number of complex issues need to be considered in developing precipitation technology. That the methods of the Harvard laboratories were transferred to industrial scale so successfully was not due to their simplicity, but to the quality and sophistication of the work carried out by Cohn and his collaborators.

The objective of the process technology is to obtain a defined uniform environment (i.e. pH, temperature, ethanol concentration, etc.) which will cause the desired protein(s) to leave solution and form a particulate solids phase which can then be readily removed by an appropriate solid–liquid separation technology.

However, to achieve this new environment, reagents must be added and temperatures adjusted. It is in making these changes that problems arise. Reagents must be added in a concentrated form but high concentrations at the point of addition (e.g. pH) can result in irreversible damage to the product protein. The addition of ethanol to water releases heat (i.e. it is an exothermic reaction); consequently it is possible to experience high local ethanol concentrations and high temperatures at the point of reagent addition both of which can cause protein denaturation.

These difficulties can be minimized by using relatively dilute reagents, with slow addition and efficient mixing. Taken together these factors make up the contacting conditions for a particular vessel or device. However, scale-up of these factors is not straightforward, with efficient mixing being particularly difficult to achieve with shear sensitive components, especially as air entrapment and foaming should be avoided to prevent surface denaturation of proteins.

Further problems emerge when we consider the nature of the particulate (solids) phase. It is now known that the initial size distribution of precipitated particles is determined by the reagent contacting conditions used and that particles can be subsequently broken down in size by shear forces experienced during mixing and on entry to centrifuges for solids recovery. The particle characteristics have a major influence on the quality of the separation achieved (e.g. on centrifugation) with large particles giving good recovery and compact solids while small particles may result in poor recoveries and loose solids. Despite these difficulties the technology for protein precipitation has advanced using specially designed batch-processing equipment with vessel capacities ranging in scale from 100 to 10 000 litres.

An alternative approach was suggested by Cohn. He envisaged a move from batch to continuous process technology and drawings of equipment for the continuous preparation of a wide range of blood and plasma products exist in his lecture papers of 1950 from Harvard Medical School. Unfortunately, Cohn died before these plans could be implemented and it was Watt in Edinburgh who later adopted the concept of continuous-flow processing to overcome many of the difficulties inherent in large-batch operations. Cold ethanol plasma fractionation by continuous-flow processing under computer control was introduced into routine use at the Scottish National Blood Transfusion Service's (SNBTS) Protein Fractionation Centre in Edinburgh in 1976 and has functioned successfully since that time. As well as providing fixed contacting of reagents with efficient heat transfer and low shear mixing, this technology has also enabled sophisticated monitoring and process control systems to be employed to assure reproducible performance. A high degree of equipment utilization can also be achieved, avoiding problems of bottlenecking at key technology limited operations (e.g. centrifugation) which beset large-batch processing. Despite these advantages, the continuous-flow processing of human plasma has still to be adopted elsewhere.

As well as being used in the manufacture of albumin and immunoglobulin products (by cold ethanol fractionation), precipitation methods are also used in the preparation of other plasma proteins (e.g. Factor VIII) where similar considerations influence the design of methods and equipment.

Advantages of precipitation

In general, precipitation is very suitable for industrial-scale processing as inexpensive reagents are readily available and experience in large-scale applications exist in a number of industries. It can be utilized to substantially reduce process volumes and to remove proteins that may otherwise interfere with more sensitive process steps such as chromatography and ultrafiltration. Protein precipitates themselves represent a very convenient means of storing intermediate materials in a compact and stable form. For example, cryoprecipitate (Factor VIII), Fraction I + II + III (IgG), Fraction II (IgG), Fraction IV4 + V (albumin) and Fraction V + VI (albumin) can all be stored as intermediate process materials in the form of frozen precipitate solids.

The cold ethanol method has the added advantage of providing a bacteriostatic environment, enabling products to be prepared free from harmful levels of bacterial lipopolysaccharides (pyrogens) without recourse to completely sterile operations. The low toxicity of ethanol and the fact that residual quantities can easily be removed are further attractions.

Disadvantages of precipitation

Disadvantages of cold ethanol fractionation include the high costs of refrigeration, the requirement for staff to work in uncomfortable conditions, and the explosion and fire risks associated with the use of a volatile organic solvent.

Precipitation is also regarded as being limited in the degree of purification that it affords, partly because of limited selectivity but also because proteins in solution are inevitably carried over within the solids phase. This latter feature results in contamination of the precipitated protein and loss of yield of the solution protein, but can partly be dealt with by washing of the solids phase. Nevertheless precipitation can provide a 20-fold increase in purification of Factor VIII with a 50-fold volume reduction in a single step (e.g. cryoprecipitation) and produces IgG of 99% purity in high yield using three-precipitation steps.

Opportunities for further development

If we return to the parameters which determine protein solubility (Table 3.2) we can see that one variable, specific ion effects, was not exploited in Cohn's Method 6. Cohn himself was well aware of this, regarding Method 6 as a relatively limited procedure. He subsequently introduced metal ions (e.g. zinc) in the development of a potentially less-denaturing procedure which became known as Method 10. This project was subsequently abandoned following Cohn's death when immunoglobulin prepared by a further development of this approach (Method 12) was found to transmit hepatitis, in contrast to cold ethanol preparations (Methods 6 and 9). Perhaps Cohn would have seen this as proof that this approach was indeed more gentle and sophisticated, regarding the problem of viral contamination as another challenge to be dealt with rather than an impediment to progress.

We believe that the full potential of precipitation has still to be achieved and that the very large number of parameters available for exploitation (Table 3.2) should, if correctly manipulated, enable a high degree of selectivity to be achieved. However, to obtain this, accurate control will be crucial and it is here that correctly designed process technology (e.g. continuous flow) will be essential. A better understanding of precipitate particle behaviour and its control is also required, allied with improved solid–liquid separation technology.

PROTEIN EXTRACTION

Background

Protein precipitates must be redissolved for further processing. Hence further opportunities exist to exploit differences in solubility behaviour amongst those proteins that make up the solids phase using the parameters already described (Table 3.2).

First, the precipitate can be washed to remove the soluble proteins which have been carried over entrapped in the solids phase, a procedure which has been applied to cryoprecipitate in Factor VIII processing.

Second, the composition of the solution used to redissolve the precipitate can be adjusted to exceed the solubility limit of selected proteins which consequently will remain undissolved and can be separated from the dissolved proteins by centrifugation or filtration. This is a process of differential extraction and can be applied for example to cryoprecipitate in Factor VIII processing and to Fraction IV4 + V in albumin processing.

Process technology

Extraction procedures do not have the problems of local reagent overshoot seen with precipitation but similar problems exist in the handling of the precipitate particles which are vulnerable to shear breakdown. Consequently, specially designed mixing systems are required to promote rapid dissolution without damaging the particles that remain insoluble and compromising their removal. Heat input and temperature control are also required as precipitates will normally be processed from the frozen state.

Opportunities for further development

The washing and differential extraction of protein precipitates is not widely used but would seem to be an area with considerable potential as it would simply be an extension to the precipitation technology already dominant in the plasma fractionation industry. However, progress in this area does require further knowledge concerning the characteristics of precipitate particles so that appropriate process equipment can be designed and controlled.

The transfer of proteins between two immiscible liquid phases (liquid–liquid extraction) is now quite widely used for the separation of biological macromolecules. However the technique has as yet made little impact in plasma fractionation.

SOLID–LIQUID SEPARATION

Background

In using their solubility characteristics to separate proteins from one another it is important to appreciate that separation is only achieved when the solid and liquid phases are parted from one another. Therefore the process of solid–liquid separation is central to the success of the operation and the conditions under which a precipitate phase has been formed (i.e. pH, temperature, etc.) must be retained within the equipment used to collect the solids. Centrifugation is most commonly used for this purpose but filtration methods are also employed.

In centrifugation, the sedimentation of particles is normally described by an equation developed from the work of Stokes in 1850:

$$V_0 = d^2(\rho_p - \rho_1)\, \omega^2 r / 18\mu$$

where V_0 = the equilibrium settling velocity of a particle, d = the particle diameter, ρ_p = the particle density, ρ_1 = the liquid density, μ = the liquid viscosity, ω = the angular velocity of rotation and r = the radius of the arc of rotation.

Although Stokes' law is based on idealized behaviour and ignores surface effects and particle–particle interactions, it does provide valuable insight into centrifugation procedures. It is especially important to note that sedimentation is a function of the particle diameter squared (d^2), causing this to be the most important of the features of the precipitate suspension which influence centrifugation.

We have already considered the factors which can influence the particle size, including reagent contacting procedures for precipitation and the effects of mixing and other process equipment in causing a reduction in particle size by shear damage. It is also possible to increase the size of protein precipitates by introducing energy at a level sufficient to cause particles to agglomerate by colliding with one another. However, to fully utilize any increase in particle size achieved, it is necessary to subsequently avoid exposing these particles to forces sufficiently strong to disrupt them.

Similar considerations apply when filtration is used instead of centrifugation, where the particle diameter is also an important parameter in the separation mechanism. Protein precipitates are made up of fine soft particles which can easily block a filter surface; consequently the form of filtration commonly used in these circumstances is depth filtration. Here the filter has a high surface area but a relatively open structure with channels much larger than particles being processed and with fine particle capture being achieved by electrostatic (charge) effects rather than simply by exclusion of the particle at the filter surface. This procedure is normally assisted by the use of filter aids, insoluble granular materials which provide a porous surface matrix which holds the larger precipitate particles to prevent them from blocking the filter; filter aids also possess adsorptive characteristics themselves which contribute to particle collection.

Process technology

Generally, there are two types of industrial centrifuge used in plasma fractionation both of which function by accumulating sedimented solids in a rotating bowl, with the feed suspension and the exiting supernatant flowing continuously until the solids capacity of the bowl is reached. At this point the machine must be run down, the solids removed by manual means and the equipment cleaned and re-assembled for further use.

The tubular bowl centrifuge (e.g. Sharples) was introduced by Cohn and is still used widely. This type of centrifuge is relatively easy to disassemble and empty but has a small solids capacity (approximately 5 kg). Temperature control is an important feature, as the desired precipitation temperature (e.g. $-5°C$) must be obtained within the centrifuge and retained throughout the operation. During centrifugation, heat is produced at the wall of the rotating bowl and from the motor and bearings. The tubular bowl centrifuge is cooled by refrigerant passing through coils in the casing surrounding the rotating bowl. However, this does not remove all of the heat being generated and it is therefore usual to site tubular bowl centrifuges in a cold area held at about $-5°C$. The limited refrigeration capacity associated with the tubular bowl centrifuge was a particularly severe constraint in continuous-flow processing and led to the development of an alternative centrifuge for this project, the refrigerated multi-chamber centrifuge (Westfalia Ltd), which was introduced in Edinburgh in the mid-1970s and is now in widespread use.

The multi-chamber centrifuge consists of up to five annular chambers fitted within a rotating cylindrical bowl. In plasma fractionation, the simplest version, the two-chamber machine is preferred as it is the easiest form to dismantle and provides solids capacities of up to 45 kg. A high refrigeration capacity is achieved by passing refrigerant through channels in the wall of the rotating bowl as well as through the casing surrounding the machine.

Depth filtration is carried out using the filter press, a device which holds flat sheets of filter material between a series of parallel stainless-steel plates. The filter press is not easily cooled and if temperature-sensitive solids are being collected, it is usually necessary to house the unit in a sub-zero area (e.g. $-5°C$).

Depth filters are best suited to the removal of small quantities of waste solids. However, there is increasing interest in their use for the collection of large-volume product solids, instead of centrifugation. This procedure requires the use of filter aids which can also introduce undesirable metal ions (e.g. aluminium), which must subsequently be removed from product fractions together with the filter aid itself. At first sight, this appears a cumbersome method to adopt but the rationale lies in the relatively high capacity of the filter press compared to centrifuges, which are limited in size by the strength of the materials of construction and the forces experienced during rotation.

This problem of centrifuge capacity is particularly acute for manufacturers using the smaller tubular bowl centrifuge to support large batch processing, as the intermittent nature of batch operation results in bottlenecking at the centrifuge. The use of centrifuges with a higher capacity (i.e. multichamber) and a higher degree of equipment utilization (e.g. by continuous-flow processing) avoids this problem.

Opportunities for further development

There are a number of areas where centrifugation may be improved. First it is probable that current equipment is not being operated under optimal conditions. It is generally assumed that centrifuges should be run at full speed to obtain maximum solids dewatering and bowl capacity. However, the higher the speed of rotation, the greater the shear force experienced by suspended particles as they enter the machine. If particle breakdown occurs as a consequence, then the benefits of a higher centrifugal force may be outweighed by the loss of performance resulting from a reduction in the particle diameter. For any combination of centrifuge and particle type, there will be an optimal centrifuge speed which will maximize performance. Such optimal operating conditions have still to be determined.

The performance of existing centrifuges would also be improved by the design of low shear entry zones to prevent particle break-up and by the development of accessories to aid solids removal. In this latter area, the potential offered by automatic solids discharge centrifuges (e.g. disc stack, scroll) remains to be achieved in plasma fractionation.

ADSORPTION/DESORPTION

Background

Proteins can be separated from one another by selective binding from solution to a solid-phase material (adsorption), either individually or in groups. Where a product protein is bound, then removal from the solid phase must be carried out subsequently (desorption), providing further selectivity.

The binding properties of the solid phase are often obtained by some form of modification to its surface chemistry or by attaching a specific chemical group (ligand). A number of mechanisms may be utilized for binding proteins, the most common being electrostatic or charge effects (ion exchange) and the use of specific binding sites (affinity chromatography). Hydrophobic, hydrophilic and covalent interactions can also occur.

Where binding occurs by a number of mechanisms simultaneously or the mechanisms(s) in a particular application is unknown, then adsorption is often described as being non-specific. Non-specific adsorption was used by Cohn and his colleagues in the 1940s in the form of depth filtration to remove lipoproteins from albumin solutions and proteolytic enzymes from immunoglobulin solutions. During the 1960s, aluminium hydroxide adsorption was introduced into Factor VIII processing to remove contaminating coagulation factors which could degrade Factor VIII and ion-exchange chromatography was introduced for the preparation of Factor IX concentrates. Affinity chromatography was introduced in 1972 with the preparation of anti-thrombin III via adsorption to heparin-agarose. Considerable development work has since been undertaken on adsorption methods and materials and these are now being used for a range of separations in plasma fractionation, a topic that will be dealt with more fully in Chapter 5.

Process technology

Processing is usually carried out batchwise either in stirred tanks or in packed beds (column chromatography); however batch tank adsorption followed by packing of the solid phase into a column for desorption is used when different process considerations apply between the adsorption and desorption stages. Where the solid and liquid phases have to be separated then either gravity sedimentation, centrifugation or filtration methods are employed.

Opportunities for further development

Adsorption methods are constrained by a number of features including lack of knowledge concerning individual protein–ligand interactions, multiple binding mechanisms occurring simultaneously, variable process performance, poor reproducibility and stability of solid-phase materials and the high cost of reagents.

Although chromatographic methods can be automated to carry out a predetermined sequence of events, process control technology has not been applied as representative changes cannot yet be monitored at the point of separation and accurate modelling of real processes has still to be achieved.

The batch mode of processing is also limiting particularly where the capacity of the solid phase is low. In these circumstances continuous operation (e.g. by fluidized bed chromatography) would have attractions but may require multi-stage operation to achieve the overall selectivity of a packed-bed process.

PRODUCT FINISHING

FORMULATION

Formulation is the conversion of biologically and pharmacologically active components into dosage forms suitable for administration to patients. In plasma fractionation this means converting various fractions, extracts or eluates from different protein separation processes into suitable dosage forms. This in turn means removing residual ethanol, removing stabilizers or contaminants from intermediate processes, adjusting salt concentrations, and adjusting protein concentrations or introducing additives required for final product stability. Traditionally, the plasma fractionation industry has used thermal technologies such as bulk freeze-drying and rotary vacuum distillation to remove ethanol from fractions, the formulation of the dried solid or concentrate being adjusted by simple reconstitution and/or dilution. Eluates and extracts (generally not containing ethanol) were more or less processed as they were or with some dilution or addition.

However, the advent of modern membrane technology, particularly microporous crossflow filtration using membranes of a defined molecular pore size (ultrafiltration) has revolutionized this operation not only in plasma fractionation but throughout the bioprocessing industries. Using ultrafiltration ethanol removal, protein concentration, salt adjustment, stabilizer addition, etc. can all be carried out in a single step in the same piece of equipment. The continuing development of membrane types and pumping systems means that this technology can be applied across a wide range of processing scales handling the most robust to the most labile of proteins.

STERILE FILTRATION AND DISPENSING

The production of pharmaceuticals for parenteral use requires the highest standards of final product sterility, and parenterals from plasma proteins are no exception. The technology used follows almost exactly that developed in the mainstream pharmaceutical industries with the exception of filter developments for protein solutions which has been a specialist area.

Since the production of sterile parenteral products has become well established, there is a tendency to take these steps for granted. However, the technology involved such as sterile room management, container and closure preparation, and product dispensing are highly developed and closely regulated. Products must be stable and recoverable in a safe form throughout their shelf life and the quality of the final product container has an important role in meeting these objectives.

FREEZE-DRYING (LYOPHILIZATION)

Several plasma products are freeze-dried in their final form mainly because of their labile nature, e.g. Factor VIII, Factor IX concentrates and intravenous immunoglobulin preparations containing residual proteolytic enzyme activity. Plasma and plasma products were amongst the first parenterals prepared using lyophilization. However, wider interest in the design of optimal freeze-drying conditions has only come with the comparatively recent increased awareness (mainly through developments in biotechnology) in proteins as macromolecular drugs. At present, improvements in freeze-drying process technology and in particular in industrial freeze-drying plant are areas of rapid development. Despite this, it is still possible to find the 'black box' approach to freeze-drying where standard protocols are applied from product to product regardless of changes in formulation and freezing characteristics.

A key development in some fractionation centres in bringing about improvements in the understanding and application of freeze-drying has been the heat treatment of lyophilized products to inactivate viral contaminants. To treat lyophilized products at high temperatures over long periods requires optimum freeze-drying conditions. We have found that product quality can be improved greatly with the application of some basic principles. These include, freezing in a manner which provides a uniform plug structure, carrying out primary drying at a temperature which ensures that drying is by sublimation alone and not partially by evaporation, and using specified time/temperature combinations in secondary drying to achieve the desired residual moisture content in the final produuct. It should also be remembered that since freeze-drying necessarily occurs after filtration and dispensing it must be carried out under the same sterility requirements.

OPPORTUNITIES FOR FURTHER DEVELOPMENT

Despite the success of membrane technology in the bioprocessing industries, membrane performance is limited by the formation of a gel layer of protein at the membrane surface. Therefore improvements in ultrafiltration performance might be achieved by preventing the formation of a gel layer, either by maintaining turbulence at the membrane surfaces (i.e. by a fluid mechanics approach), or through the development of membranes with low protein binding characteristics (i.e. by changes in the membrane polymer-surface chemistry).

The improvements in freeze-drying plant have not been matched by imrovements in process control during lyophilization. In general, freeze-drying protocols are still based on retrospective measurements of temperature from a small number of product probes with no feedback from product to machine. The use of more sophisticated data gathering and control systems would allow improved drying, more efficient use of plant and easier (and so less expensive) scale up from small laboratory or pilot freeze driers to production plant.

VIRUS INACTIVATION

The transmission of viruses by the use of untreated human blood products has made the safety of clinical products a major issue in plasma fractionation. The blood transfusion community worldwide has been well aware of these problems and testing all donations for the presence of human immunodeficiency virus (HIV) and hepatitis is required practice. However, test systems have a finite sensitivity and cannot detect the presence of viruses in the period between infection and the appearance of a sufficient concentration of specific antibodies or antigens; nor can test systems detect as yet unidentified or undiscovered viruses which is just how HIV infection arose in blood products. There is a need therefore, in addition to identification and screening procedures, for inactivation procedures also, as part of an overall strategy. There are several virus-inactivation methods being used currently in the preparation of plasma products.

HEATING IN SOLUTION

Albumin products have been heated in solution at 60°C for 10 h ('pasteurisation') for over 40 years with an outstanding safety record against a range of potentially infective agents. Albumin can be stabilized relatively easily for heating in solution by using low concentrations of non-toxic additives (sodium caprylate, sodium acetyltryptophanate). Since the final product form of albumin is as a solution, the heating can be performed as a terminal step in the sealed final product container, which eliminates all possibility of accidental infection by contaminated equipment or other batches. The use of a heat inactivation method in this way is also advantageous in that it is relatively simple to validate that each container in a batch of product has been subjected to the correct time/temperature combination and a record can be kept for each pasteurization treatment.

There are no simple stabilizing formulations for the heating in solution of products which, unlike albumin, contain labile biological activities. Human Factor VIII activity, for example, can only be stabilized against pasteurization at 60°C for 10 h by the addition of high concentrations of carbohydrate and glycine. However, such formulations cannot be used for final products and extra processing is required to remove the stabilizers after heat treatment.

HEATING IN THE LYOPHILIZED (FREEZE-DRIED) STATE

Several plasma products, for example coagulation factors, are lyophilized preparations. The development of appropriate formulations and freeze-drying cycles has enabled lyophilized coagulation factor preparations to be heated at high temperatures for prolonged periods (80°C for 72 h) in their final product form with good recoveries across the heating step. Products heated in this manner have been shown to be potentially very safe from virus infection and because the heat treatment can be applied as a terminal step they have the additional safety advantage of there being no possibility of recontamination.

CHEMICAL TREATMENTS

Several chemical treatments have been used as virus inactivation procedures in the manufacture of plasma products. These include the treatment of bulk intermediate solutions with β-propiolactone in combination
with UV irradiation and a similar bulk intermediate step using an organic
solvent, tri(n-butyl)phosphate (TNBP) together with a detergent usually
Tween-80 or sodium deoxycholate. This latter method has been evaluated
extensively in blood product applications showing good yield and safety
characteristics. However, non-lipid enveloped viruses are resistant to
TNBP/detergent, which limits the range of viruses against which this
method is effective.

All methods which use potentially toxic reagents require considerable
extra processing steps to remove these reagents.

PROCESS DESIGN

There are important process design issues to be considered in establishing
virus inactivation procedures. These issues arise from the fundamentally
different nature of the current inactivation methods, i.e. physical (heat) and
chemical, and the different stages in a process where virus inactivation can
be introduced, i.e. as an intermediate step or as a terminal step. For example,
it is not a simple matter to ensure for a bulk batch treatment method that the
same degree of chemical contacting takes place either from batch to batch or
within a batch. The effects of scale are also important considerations in
accurately reproducing the inactivation process at laboratory level (scale
down), for example to calibrate its effectiveness using model viruses. A non-
invasive method applied to final products can be carried out on one vial or
many vials with equal validity.

The possible risk of process failure should also be considered when designing a virus-inactivation step. For example, when virus inactivation is
carried out as an intermediate step, the product is at risk of contamination
downstream of the inactivation procedure but with a terminal inactivation
step (i.e. carried out on the product in its final sealed container) the risk of
batch failure through subsequent contamination does not exist.

OPPORTUNITIES FOR FURTHER DEVELOPMENT

Since virus inactivation processes are relatively new for most plasma products other than albumin, this field remains open for developments. The
challenge in devising new virus-inactivation strategies will be to adhere to
the best design principles. This may require the development of chemical or
combined physical and chemical processes which can be used in the final
products. Near terminal inactivation procedures which might be applied in

a continuous-flow mode during dispensing such as irradiation or ohmic heating might also prove fruitful areas of work. Alternatively, one could meet the prime design criterion of avoiding all possibility of cross-contamination during processing by inactivating all plasma before it enters the plasma fractionation plant. In selecting a procedure, concepts of risk analysis may be employed to assess the overall security associated with different options.

FUTURE DEVELOPMENTS

There can be no doubting that the rapid growth of the bioindustries, particularly the development of macromolecular (protein) drugs, has had a marked effect on the plasma fractionation industry. This effect has been seen mainly in the areas of Regulatory affairs and process technology and it is our view that these trends will continue.

REGULATORY ISSUES

As plasma fractionation continues to mature from a largely isolated and specialist activity to become fully integrated into the pharmaceutical and process sector, there will be a greater input from the disciplines of pharmaceutical engineering and biochemical engineering. Inspection and control, which at the moment are slanted heavily towards the biological nature of the substances being manufactured, will have a greater engineering content involving the design, commissioning, validation, routine operation and suitability of process plant.

In a related field, the increased use of computing in process control, process monitoring and data gathering (both analytical and manufacturing) will require the validation of software used in the process industries.

Feedstock control and the licensing of donor centres together with their products and services other than plasma will also be a significant area of future Regulatory activity in the UK and elsewhere.

Virus inactivation has become an increasingly important feature of plasma fractionation and for the production of pharmaceutical proteins from other biological sources. However, it remains relatively unregulated with different centres measuring virus inactivation or elimination using different techniques and organisms. A standard panel of viruses should be required for testing in a standardized manner and that testing should be monitored by the respective national control authorities.

There may also be regulatory requirements for further information on product pharmacology, especially in the development of new products. Studies would be required to demonstrate that a new product has enough potential to merit clinical evaluation and to identify the physicochemical properties of the protein that could affect its performance as a drug and influence the development of a safe efficacious dosage form.

PROCESS TECHNOLOGY

Advances in process techniques being developed throughout industry may find particular application in plasma fractionation. This is already happening in the development of centrifuges, freeze-drying plant and membrane processes and is likely to become more prevalent as biotechnology moves towards greater use of industrial equipment. For example, much of the thinking on separation technology in this field is dominated by attempting to scale-up highly-selective laboratory techniques, whereas significant advances are more likely to be made by improving the selectivity of methods which already have good scale-up characteristics. The ever-improving aqueous two-phase (liquid–liquid) extraction of proteins is an example of this approach. If plasma protein separation can be established in stable immiscible phases, then a whole field of already vastly successful industrial separation technology and plant will be opened up to plasma fractionation.

Another major area of future process development is expected to result from increased Regulatory activity, in that new plant and processes will have to comply with greater levels of control and operate under increased Regulatory constraints.

PRODUCT RANGE

Human plasma contains a large number of proteins of potential therapeutic importance and yet few of these are established in clinical use. To demonstrate the therapeutic value of new plasma protein products they must be tested clinically, but the testing of these products has in most cases been outweighed by the risk of infection. However, recent advances in virus inactivation techniques, allied to developments in separation technology and improvements in Regulatory control, has changed this situation dramatically and a wide range of new plasma products is likely to emerge for clinical evaluation over the coming years.

FURTHER READING

Bell, D.J., Hoare, M. and Dunnill, P. (1983) The formation of protein precipitates and their centrifugal recovery. *Advances in Biochemical Engineering* (Ed. A. Fiechter), **26**, pp. 1–72. Springer-Verlag, New York.
Chase, H.A. (1988) Adsorption separation processes for protein purification. In: *Advances in Biotechnological Processes*, **8**, pp. 159–204. Alan R. Liss, New York.
Cheryan, M. (1986) *Ultrafiltration Handbook*. Technomic, Lancaster.

Cuthbertson, B. *et al.* (1991) Viral contamination of human plasma and procedures for preventing virus transmission by plasma products. In: *Blood Separation and Plasma Fractionation* (Ed. J.R. Harris). Wiley–Liss, London.

DeSain, C. (1990) *Drug, Device and Diagnostic Manufacturing. The Ultimate Resource Handbook.* Interpharm Press, Buffalo Grove.

Finlayson, J.S. and Aronson, D.L. (1979–80) Therapeutic plasma fractions and plasma fractionation. *Seminars in Thrombosis and Haemostasis,* **6**, 1–139.

Foster, P.R. *et al.* (1986) A process control system for the fractional precipitation of human plasma proteins. *Journal of Chemical Technology and Biotechnology,* **36**, 461–466.

McIntosh, R.V. and Foster, P.R. (1990) The effect of solution formulation on the stability and surface interactions of Factor VIII during plasma fractionation. *Transfusion Science,* **II**, 55–66.

McIntosh, R.V. *et al.* (1990) Freezing and thawing plasma. In *Developments in Hematology and Immunology,* (Eds Smit-Sibinga, C. Th. *et al.*), **24**, pp. 11–24. Kluwer, Boston.

Meltzer, T.H. (Ed.) (1987) *Filtration in the Pharmaceutical Industry.* Marcel Dekker, New York.

Pennell, R.B. (1960) Fractionation and isolation of purified components by precipitation methods. In: *The Plasma Proteins* (Ed. F.W. Putnam), **1**, pp. 9–50. Academic Press, New York.

Stryker, M.H. *et al.* (1985) Blood fractionation: proteins. In: *Advances in Biotechnological Processes,* **4**, pp. 275–336. Alan R. Liss, New York.

Williams, N.A. and Polli, G.P. (1984) The lyophilisation of pharmaceuticals: a literature review. *Journal of Parenteral Science & Technology,* **38**, 48–59.

4 Biotechnological Approaches to the Provision of Products

S. MOORE and A.J. MacLEOD

INTRODUCTION

The rapid development of recombinant DNA technology in the last decade has revolutionized the future prospects for producing therapeutic proteins which, until recently, have been produced by fractionation of naturally occurring sources, especially human blood plasma. In this chapter we will outline the principles behind the currently available techniques for producing proteins by recombinant DNA technology with particular emphasis on the use of transfected mammalian cells in culture.

A major level of the control of protein synthesis occurs at the transcriptional level, thus an understanding of the basic mechanisms of both transcription and translation is essential in order to design an expression system. It is clearly desirable that for consideration as the basis of a process for the production of a therapeutic protein, a cell should be capable of high-level expression of biologically active product which is correctly folded and has the appropriate post-translational modifications such as glycosylation, amino acid modifications and specific proteolytic cleavages. In addition, the feasibility of producing an acceptable product, including cell cultivation, downstream processing and ease of satisfying regulatory requirements, at an economic cost, must be taken fully into account. These aspects of the various options are summarized in Table 4.1. On the basis of this type of analysis, a general consensus has emerged that for the immediate future mammalian cells cultured *in vitro* are the system of choice for production of proteins for clinical use. Therefore, the first section of this chapter will be devoted to giving a basic outline of the salient points of the main transcription, translation and production systems with particular reference to mammalian cells. This description is necessarily brief and the reader is referred to the further reading at the end of this chapter for more detailed information.

Plasma and Recombinant Blood Products in Medical Therapy
Edited by C.V. Prowse. Published 1992 by John Wiley & Sons Ltd

Table 4.1 Summary of the merits of various systems for the production of therapeutic proteins

Expression system	Advantages	Disadvantages
Bacteria	Established large-scale production technology Rapid production of large amounts of proteins Low production costs	Random folding forms product as insoluble intracellular granules No secondary modifications Incomplete proteolytic cleavage Cellular components highly antigenic and pyrogenic: a very high degree of product purification required
Yeast	Established large-scale production technology Rapid production of large amounts of protein Low production costs	Pattern of secondary modification very different from that found on mammalian proteins Cellular components highly antigenic: a very high degree of product purification required
Mammalian cells	Large-scale production technology becoming generally available Authentic native protein produced with a relatively low antigenicity	Complex operation of many large-scale production systems Complex medium Relatively high operating costs Risk that contaminating microorganisms may be pathogenic: require stringent removal/inactivation steps in downstream processing
Transgenic animals	Authentic native protein produced with a relatively low antigenicity Product harvest without comprising production system	Production in complex medium requiring a very high degree of purification Difficult to organize animal husbandry in compliance with GMP requirements Risk that microorganisms infecting the animals may be pathogenic in man: require stringent removal/inactivation steps in downstream processing Relatively long delay before large amounts of protein can be produced

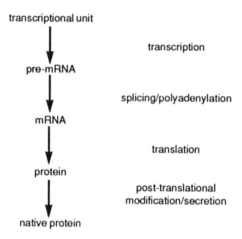

Fig. 4.1. Sequential steps in protein synthesis

BASIC PRINCIPLES

Figure 4.1 shows the 'basic dogma' of molecular biology – the sequential steps in protein synthesis starting with the transcriptional unit.

TRANSCRIPTION

A general model of an actively transcribed eukaryotic transcriptional unit (gene) is shown in Figure 4.2. Promoter elements are found in the region −40 to −200 base pairs (bp) from the transcriptional start site and serve as binding sites for transacting transcription proteins which are necessary for the formation of a pre-initiation complex incorporating RNA polymerase-II. Many different transcriptional proteins have been identified. Some are found in most cell types while others have a more restricted range. Furthermore, promoters can differ considerably in their structure when comparing different

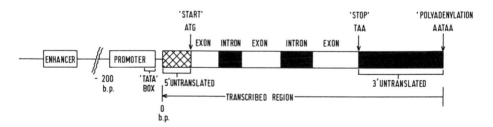

Fig. 4.2. Model of an actively transcribed eukaryotic transcriptional unit (gene)

transcriptional units and as a consequence binding sites for particular transcriptional proteins may be absent in one promoter but present in another. In
this way, the cell specific regulation of gene expression can be achieved.

A general feature of the promoter regions of actively transcribed eukaryotic genes is the so-called TATA box. This is a highly-conserved sequence
which occurs 25–35 bp upstream from the transcriptional start site and is
important for the accurate positioning of transcription initiation. Mutations
in the TATA box sequence drastically reduce the rate of transcription.

Enhancers serve a similar function to promoter sequences except that they
are often located at a considerable distance (up to 10 000 bp, i.e. 10 kb)
upstream/downstream or even, in one or two cases, within the transcribed
region itself. Enhancers can vary in their tissue specificity and in their relative strengths. The human cytomegalovirus (CMV) enhancer is one of the
strongest known.

The polyadenylation signal, AATAAA, is important for the correct processing of the primary RNA transcript. Cleavage of the primary RNA transcript occurs 15–30 bp downstream from the polyadenylation signal and
subsequently addition of a poly(A) tail of approximately 250 residues occurs. Mutations in the poly(A) signal sequence result in reduction or aboli-
tion of the 3' end formation. Naturally-occurring variants of the AATAAA
sequence may be intentional 'weak' poly(A) sites to restrict mRNA production, e.g. in 'housekeeping' genes where low level transcription is required.

Untranslated regions vary considerably in length from as little as 10 bp at
the 5' end to many kilobases (kb) at the 3' end. The function of these regions
is not clearly understood but in the case of the 3' region may include
sequences which regulate the stability of mRNA, e.g. AU rich sequences
have been shown to confer instability on mRNA and are present in some
transiently-expressed genes.

TRANSLATION

When designing an expression system for producing plasma proteins we are
primarily concerned with expressing proteins which are secreted from the
cell. It is therefore important to consider some of the essential aspects of
secretory protein biosynthesis so that an optimum system for production of
biologically-active protein can be devised.

The initial stages of secretory protein biosynthesis occur while the ribosome is in the cytosol. An N-terminal signal sequence of approximately 16–
30 amino acid residues is present in most secretory proteins and functions to
direct insertion of the nascent polypeptide into the membrane of the endoplasmic reticulum (ER). Protein synthesis continues with the ribosome
bound to the ER membrane. On emergence into the ER lumen, the signal
sequence is cleaved and peptide elongation continues until synthesis is complete and the ribosome released. The newly-synthesized protein then passes

into the ER lumen where it is subjected to maturation, sorting and transportation processes before secretion from the cell. The four principal processes in maturation for many secretory proteins are:

- formation of disulphide bonds necessary for stabilizing tertiary structure
- accurate folding
- specific proteolytic cleavages
- glycosylation

These modifications are necessary for the protein to achieve a functional form.

Disulphide bonding occurs in the ER lumen, is often initiated during elongation and is subject to enzyme catalysis to allow rapid attainment of a thermodynamically stable conformation. Improperly folded proteins are prevented from leaving the ER. In some cases this is due to binding to ER membrane proteins such as BIP (heavy-chain binding protein).

Many secretory proteins are initially synthesized as a pro-protein and require the action of specific endoproteases which cleave at a specific site(s) within the polypeptide to generate active, mature molecules. This process usually occurs at a late stage in maturation, e.g. pro-insulin is converted to insulin in the secretory vesicles.

Glycosylation is an important aspect of the biosynthesis of secretory proteins which contain one or more carbohydrate groups. Correct glycosylation is often required for the attainment of the native conformation of the protein and hence its biological activity. Furthermore, it may be important for secretion of the protein and an increasing resistance to proteolytic degradation and hence increasing the half-life of the molecule. Glycosylation is classified into two main types: (i) O-linked to serine or threonine residues; (ii) N-linked to asparagine. The initial stage of N-glycosylation occurs co-translationally in the ER lumen. Subsequent processing and addition of O-glycosylation occurs sequentially via a vesicular transport mechanism in discrete compartments of the Golgi apparatus and is catalysed by specific glycosyl transferases and glycosidases. When contemplating production of therapeutic proteins by recombinant DNA techniques, it is important to avoid incorrect glycosylation which can result in highly antigenic structures being present on the protein, e.g. while glycosylation can occur in yeast cells it is not necessarily equivalent to that of the native protein.

CONSTRUCTING AN EXPRESSION SYSTEM

SOURCE OF CODING SEQUENCE

The first stage in the construction of an expression system is to obtain the appropriate DNA coding sequences for insertion into the expression vector.

It is almost certain that for a protein intended for therapeutic use, the gene will already have been cloned and sequenced and considerable information on the structure of the protein will be available.

It is important to distinguish between genomic DNA and cDNA because the use of one or other source may be inappropriate in a particular circumstance. Genomic DNA clones are isolated by screening genomic libraries. These are prepared by restriction endonuclease cleavage of total genomic DNA of the organism. The resulting fragments are inserted into a cloning vector derived from either bacterial plasmid or bacteriophage sequences and cloned by transformation of a host cell, usually E. coli. Clones containing the sequence(s) of interest are identified in the library by probing, often with a specific nucleotide probe derived from the published nucleotide sequence. In genomic clones, it is likely that the 5' untranscribed region may be present. This will contain the natural promoter sequences which may not be capable of strong transcriptional activation and/or may show specificity for a limited range of cell types. The 3' untranslated sequences may contain sequences which adversely affect the processing and stability of mRNA. It is likely, therefore, that for construction of a high-level expression system these sequences will be replaced by sequences known to direct high-level expression in the cell type to be used. Furthermore, for many genes, the genomic sequence may be too large to be accommodated in currently-available expression vectors, e.g. Factor VIII gene is 186 kb in size. In addition, multiple transcripts may be possible for genomic DNA resulting from alternative splicing.

cDNA clones are obtained from total cell mRNA isolated from a cell which expresses the desired protein by reverse transcription using the enzyme reverse transcriptase. Second strand synthesis is then performed and resulting double-stranded DNA cloned and the desired clones isolated by probing the library. The advantage of using cDNA clones is that intron and untranscribed sequences are not present thus the complete coding sequence often will be available as a single clone of manageable size, e.g. Factor VIII is ca. 9 kb in length and can therefore be comfortably accommodated in current expression vectors. More recently, the polymerase chain reaction (PCR) technique for amplifying specific DNA and RNA sequences in complex mixtures (e.g. genomic DNA digests or total cell RNA) has been used. This can simplify the isolation of desired sequences.

CHOICE OF EXPRESSION SYSTEM

It is clear from the above outline of the biosynthesis of secretory proteins that the type of cell chosen for an expression system must be capable of high-level expression of biologically-active product which is correctly folded and has the appropriate post-translational modifications, i.e. correct glycosylation, amino acid modifications where appropriate and specific proteolytic cleavages.

TECHNIQUES FOR THE EXPRESSION OF CLONED GENES

A basic requirement for expression of cloned genes in mammalian cells is the availability of a transfection procedure for introducing the gene into the cell to obtain expression. A number of transfection procedures are available of which the calcium phosphate technique is the most widely used. In this procedure calcium phosphate is co-precipitated with the DNA to be transfected and the precipitate introduced into the cell culture flask and allowed to settle onto the cells. DNA is taken up by a proportion of cells. Expression of transfected DNA occurs in two main forms: (i) transient and (ii) stable expression.

Transient expression of transfected DNA may be detected within a few hours and reaches a maximum from approximately 24–48 h after transfection, depending on the cell type. At this stage, DNA has been taken up by the nucleus but has not become integrated into the host cell genome. Transient expression is particularly useful in the initial stages of development of an expression system for optimizing transfection procedures and for analysing the efficiency of control sequences, e.g. promoters/enhancers, in a particular cell type, because results are quickly obtained. Reporter genes are often used in these initial studies and are usually genes coding for readily-assayed enzymes not found naturally in mammalian cells. The most widely used reporter is the CAT (chloramphenicol acetyltransferase) gene. CAT activity is readily assayed by measuring acetylation of ^{14}C-chloramphenicol substrate and detecting the products by thin-layer chromatography.

In order to produce usable quantities of recombinant protein, it is necessary to isolate cells which stably express the desired product. This can be achieved by using viral expression vectors such as bovine papilloma virus (BPV). In this case, a high copy number of the transfected vector (up to several hundred copies) is stably maintained in the cell as episomal, non-integrated DNA. However, construction and use of BPV vectors is somewhat more complex than the more generally used approach of achieving stable integration of transfected DNA into the host genome.

Stable integration of transfected DNA occurs in a small percentage of cells, therefore some means of isolating the stably transfected cells from non-transfected cells is essential. This is achieved by transfecting a dominant selectable marker gene driven by a eukaryotic promoter/enhancer, for example the gene for neomycin or hygromycin resistance, along with the gene to be expressed. The appropriate selection agent is incorporated into the culture medium following transfection and resistant cells isolated as clones. The selectable marker gene can be incorporated into the same vector as the gene to be expressed or incorporated into a separate vector which is co-transfected with the marker gene. In the latter case, an excess of gene to be expressed over marker gene is used to ensure that the majority of the cells selected will also have stably integrated and expressed DNA coding for the desired protein. This simplifies screening of clones.

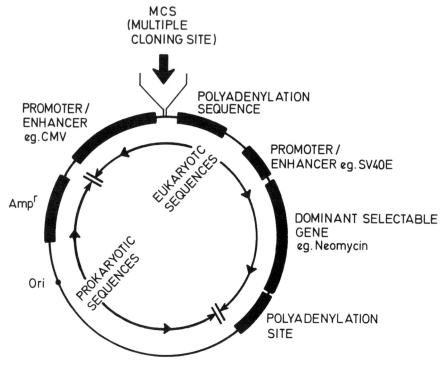

Fig. 4.3. Typical expression vector used for mammalian cells

Figure 4.3 shows the essential features of a typical expression vector used for mammalian cells. The plasmid contains prokaryotic sequences, origin of replication and antibiotic resistance gene (usually ampicillin) to allow propagation and cloning in a bacterial host (usually *E. coli*). These sequences are important to the construction and preparative isolation of the plasmid. The eukaryotic sequences contain a multiple cloning site (MCS) immediately downstream from a eukaryotic promoter/enhancer sequence, e.g. SV40E or human cytomegalovirus. Coding sequences for the gene to be expressed are inserted into the MCS using an appropriate restriction site. A dominant selectable gene is also shown but as noted above, this can be co-transfected on a separate construct. Finally, in the construction of an expression vector, it is important to ensure that the appropriate signal peptide and poly-adenylation sequences are present.

INCREASING THE COPY NUMBER OF THE TRANSFECTED GENE

In addition to choosing the optimum promoter/enhancer/cell type combination to obtain high-level expression of transfected genes, it may be possible to increase expression still further by increasing the number of copies of the recombinant gene. It is often found that the level of expression of a gene is roughly proportional to the copy number.

The technique of *gene amplification* relies on the naturally-occurring random gene-amplification events which occur in proliferating cells, probably as a result of errors in DNA replication. A feature of gene amplification is that the region of the genome which is amplified in one event is often >1000 kb, therefore adjacent genes will be co-amplified by the same event. For example, if appropriate concentrations of some cytotoxic drugs are introduced into cell cultures, clones can often be isolated which have an increased drug resistance due to amplification of an endogenous gene coding for an enzyme which confers resistance to the drug. The most widely known example of an amplifiable gene is that of the dihydrofolate reductase (DHFR) gene, whose product is specifically inhibited by methotrexate.

The practical consequence of the above is that if an amplifiable gene (e.g. DHFR) and the gene for a recombinant protein are present on the same transfected plasmid, an amplification event which amplifies the amplifiable gene will also amplify the recombinant gene. Furthermore, amplification can be repeated by exposure of resistant cells to even higher concentrations of the drug. In the case of DHFR, practical considerations have largely limited its use to Chinese hamster ovary (CHO) *dhfr⁻* cells which have no endogenous DHFR activity. More recently, other amplifiable marker genes have been used, e.g. glutamine synthetase (GS) and adenosine deaminase (ADA). Use of these markers is possible in cells which express endogenous activity, i.e. they can be used as dominant selectable genes and are thus potentially usable in many different cell lines.

PROTEIN ENGINEERING

The advent of recombinant DNA technology has revolutionized the study of protein structure–function relationships. It is now possible to use a variety of techniques to alter the base sequences in cloned genes and subsequently to express the gene to analyze the effect of the introduced mutations. This is often called 'reverse genetics'.

Mutations can be classified into three general types:

- *point mutations* where specific bases are changed
- *deletions* where sections of the gene are removed
- *insertions* where additional sequences not found in the native gene are introduced

Point mutations

There are a number of available techniques to introduce point mutations. A commonly used technique is the uracil method (see Figure 4.4). In this

mutated
nucleotide

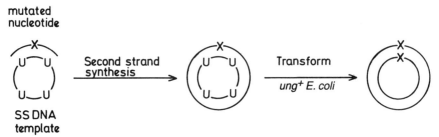

SS DNA
template

Fig. 4.4. The uracil method

procedure, single-stranded DNA is prepared, using a phage or phagemid technique, in a strain of *E. coli* deficient in the enzymes dUTPase (*dut⁻*) and uracil-*N*-glycosylase (*ung⁻*). These cells contain elevated levels of dUTP which competes with TTP for incorporation into DNA. Lack of the uracil-*N*-glycosylase repair system, which normally removes uracil from DNA, allows uracil to be incorporated into DNA. Uracil is not mutagenic. An oligonucleotide containing the required mismatch is hybridized to the single-stranded uracil containing DNA and the complementary strand synthesized *in vitro* by primer extension using DNA polymerase and dATP, dCTP, TTP and dGTP. UTP is not included in the reaction mix. The double-stranded DNA obtained is then used to transform an *ung⁺ E. coli* strain. The enzyme uracil-*N*-glycosylase removes uracil from the template strand. These are lethal lesions, probably because they block DNA synthesis of the affected strand. As a result, the progeny DNA molecules are largely derived from the second strand, i.e. the strand containing the desired point mutation. Using this procedure >50% mutagenesis can be obtained thus mutants are easily identified by sequencing plasmid DNA from a small number of clones.

Deletions

Segments of DNA can be deleted by techniques which include excizing with appropriate restriction endonucleases followed by religation and also by exonuclease digestion.

Insertions

Sequences can be inserted at an appropriate site usually by restriction digestion and ligation.

The availability of techniques for producing proteins with specific modifications is of considerable importance for the future production of therapeutic products because we are no longer tied to using naturally-occurring proteins. As our knowledge of the relationship between protein structure and function increases, it will become increasingly possible to synthesize recombinant proteins with desired specific properties for therapeutic use. Studies of the effects of varying the amino acid sequence at the active site of α_1-antitrypsin (α_1-protease inhibitor) provide an excellent example of the possibilities of protein engineering and particularly how very small sequence alterations can have a marked effect on protein function. It has been shown that methionine-358 (Met^{358}) plays a crucial role in the inhibitory activity of α_1-antitrypsin. Site-specific mutagenesis studies in which Met^{358} is replaced by different amino acid residues have been reported. The results show, for example, that a Met^{358} to Arg results in the loss of anti-elastase activity and a marked increase in the antithrombin activity of the protein while a Met^{358} to Leu change produces a potent inhibitor of neutrophil proteases, elastase and cathepsin G. Both these variants are thought to have considerable therapeutic potential.

Studies on the production of recombinant Factor VIII provide a good example of how deletion of a section of the native protein can improve the product yield. It has been shown that deletion of the B coding region of Factor VIII cDNA results in an increased yield from transfected cells possibly due to reduced retention of the product by proteins on the wall of the endoplasmic reticulum.

PRODUCTION

Genes for human plasma proteins have been expressed in members of almost every category of organism, ranging from bacteria and yeast to plants and whole mammals and in *in vitro* cultures of cells derived from members of the more complex multicellular groups. Many of these systems offer little prospect for development into processes for routine production of therapeutic proteins for use in humans but a few are being, or have been, vigorously developed for precisely this application.

BACTERIA

The first recombinant DNA systems to be developed used bacteria, notably *E. coli*, as the expression system and the initial success in this led to confident assertions that production of therapeutic proteins from plasma would soon be achieved. Systems using bacteria had the advantage from the start that a well-established technology already existed for very large-scale processing in compliance with pharmaceutical manufacturing requirements. This used simple nutrient medium in basic culture vessels which combined to give low production costs. Their rapid growth meant that newly constructed recombinant organisms could be expanded to large-scale production relatively rapidly and they could accumulate the recombinant protein to a high proportion of their total biomass, thus substantial quantities of the product could be synthesized in a short time.

However, the use of bacterial systems for the production of recombinant DNA proteins also had several disadvantages. It was obvious from the start that if the products from these systems were to be used safely in routine clinical practice then an exceptionally high degree of purification would be required to avoid antigenic and pyrogenic complications caused by bacterial macromolecules and this had a substantial adverse effect on the yield of the product from the overall process. Further complications were introduced by the discovery that bacteria could not assemble mammalian proteins into their native form, in particular disulphide bonds were made at random and the result was the production of insoluble inclusion bodies of protein that accumulated within the bacterial cell. In some cases this phenomenon could be exploited by making the isolation and thorough washing of the inclusion bodies the first step in the downstream processing of the protein. This reduced dramatically the load of bacterial material that the downstream processing had to remove. The downstream processing, however, had to include resolubilization of the protein by denaturation of the inclusion bodies and controlled renaturation into its native form which introduced the risk that many slightly different structural analogues could be generated and that there could be an immune response to these novel structures. Thus there was still a requirement for exceptionally rigorous downstream processing with the consequent imposition of a penalty on yield. Having produced and purified protein, however, there was still a problem with production of most human plasma proteins of clinical interest in that bacteria were incapable of making secondary modifications to proteins, such as glycosylation, which could have profound effects on the antigenicity or pharmacokinetics *in vivo*. Thus although bacterial systems have been used with notable success in the production of insulin, the production of larger, more complex, proteins has been based on systems using more complex organisms.

YEASTS

Yeasts, among the most basic eukaryotes, have been used successfully for the production of recombinant proteins and have the particular advantage over bacteria that they are capable of organizing the assembly and, if necessary, the glycosylation of mammalian proteins, although (as explained above) the pattern is not similar to that found on authentic mammalian proteins and is in general characterized by a much higher degree of glycosylation in proteins secreted by yeast. Consequently, recombinant yeasts have been used particularly as a basis for the production of human albumin which, since it is not a glycoprotein, avoids the problem of hyperglycosylation.

MAMMALIAN CELLS

Mammalian cells have the advantage, for the *in vitro* production of human proteins, of being more closely related to the cells and tissue that produce the proteins *in vivo* than are the cells of organisms from other families. Thus, the proteins would be correctly assembled, but although secondary modification would be done, details – especially of glycosylation – would undoubtedly vary depending on the species from which the cell was derived. However, this variation need not be large and the widespread adoption of CHO cells as expression systems has been based in part on close similarity between the pattern of glycosylation of the recombinant protein produced in this system and that of the native human protein. Another category of secondary modification that has been shown to be carried out successfully in mammalian cells is the γ-carboxylation of glutamic acid residues in the prothrombin group of coagulation factors. Mammalian cells also have the advantage that it may be possible to immortalize normal cells producing a protein of interest, either by infection with a transforming virus or by fusion with an intrinsically immortal cell line such as a myeloma. The most spectacularly successful example of this approach, which avoids many of the complications of recombinant DNA techniques but does involve very extensive screening and selection of the resulting hybrids, has been the development of hybridomas synthesizing monoclonal antibodies.

Mammalian cells can be grown on a scale sufficient to produce several kilograms of protein in compliance with pharmaceutical manufacturing requirements. Although they do not grow as rapidly as bacteria or yeasts, they do still grow sufficiently rapidly to generate a production scale culture in a relatively short time. However, compared with the bacterial or yeast systems there is still very little experience of large-scale operation of mammalian cell cultures. The nutrient medium required by mammalian cells is complex, often with undefined components, and is difficult to sterilize which results in high basic operating costs. The cells do not grow under normal conditions to the densities achieved in bacterial systems and the product only accumulates to a low level in the culture supernatant. This situation has stimulated a great deal of interest in mammalian cell-culture process intensification and many novel approaches have been proposed.

TRANSGENIC ANIMALS

The use of genetically-modified whole animals, transgenic animals, for expression of human proteins, has been shown to be technically possible and secretion of the protein into the milk facilitates separation of the product from the synthesizing system without compromising continued production. Many of the advantages of using mammalian cells apply also to using whole mammals, the protein produced would be expected to be essentially the native protein with the correct pattern of secondary modification. However, there would be severe difficulties in the way of organizing such a system to ensure production in compliance with current pharmaceutical manufacturing requirements and a limitation on the utility of systems based on whole animals is the length of time required to expand production from the original transgenic individual, which would depend on the reproductive cycle of the animal and the ability to clone embryos.

CELL-CULTURE TECHNOLOGY

The technology used for recombinant DNA protein production using bacteria or yeasts is based on the well-established batch or fed-batch fermentation systems developed for brewing or for antibiotic production. This approach is sufficiently productive and economical that there is little incentive for manufacturers to invest in the more complex and costly equipment that would be required for more sophisticated methods such as continuous culture which would also introduce complications as regards maintaining strain stability in rapidly growing organisms over a prolonged period of time and which may increase the risk of process failure through contamination.

Mammalian cells can be cultured *in vitro* in batch or fed-batch culture systems directly analogous to those used for bacterial or yeast cultures. However, in clear distinction from bacterial or yeast cultures, with mammalian cells continuous culture does offer a basis for process intensification leading to significant increases in productivity and better economy of operation. The consequence of this has been the array of culture systems that have been designed to intensify animal cell culture to achieve these ends. In general, processes fall into one of two categories depending on whether or not the cells are distributed more or less homogeneously by suspension in the culture medium. Some cell lines, notably hybridomas derived from lymphoid tissue, are able to grow freely in suspension either as clumps or as individual cells. Other cell lines need a surface to which they can adhere before they can proliferate and in these cases a solid base can be provided by the use of micro-carrier beads which provide a very large surface area for cell attachment and which can be suspended in the culture medium. Whether a cell line is free-growing or adherent is usually a fixed characteristic but with some it is possible to select variants with one or the other feature.

A further variation applicable to either free-growing or to adherent cells, is encapsulation which serves to confine the cells within beads that can then be suspended in the nutrient medium in the same way as micro-carriers. This is a hybrid system having the cells packed in beads that are distributed homogeneously in the culture medium. The alternative to the homogeneous suspension system is to have the cells packed at close to tissue density with an arrangement for supply of oxygen and other nutrients and removal of metabolic waste products. The hollow fibre bioreactor is a familiar version of this type of reactor in which the cells are packed around microporous fibres in a cartridge, the nutrient medium being circulated through the lumens of the fibres. The cell product is retained in the space around the cells where it concentrates and from where it can be tapped off periodically. In other systems with the same basic approach, the cell product may be released into the recirculating stream of nutrient medium but the essential feature is still that the cells are collected at great density in packed beds in one part of the system and are not distributed homogeneously throughout it.

With all culture systems, arrangements have to be made to monitor and, if necessary, control critical parameters (such as temperature, pH and dissolved oxygen content of the nutrient medium using on-line probes) and others including the levels of important nutrients such as glucose and glutamine and the level of the cell product using off-line methods. Suspension culture techniques have the advantage that, with careful process design, all of the cells are maintained in the same environment which can be characterized, and representative samples of cells can be taken to establish directly such features as viability and the proportion still synthesizing the cell product, a measure of the cell-line stability. In packed-cell systems, on the other hand, concentration gradients of nutrients and of cell products must exist within the cell mass so that even if probes could be located amongst the cells they would report only the conditions at their tip. In fact in these systems the probes are located outside the cell mass so that much important information about the culture has to be inferred, and even then represents an averaging out of the conditions around individual cells. As it is not possible to extract samples of the cells for routine examination in the course of a culture, their condition cannot be monitored. The effect of the concentration gradients on the cells can be reduced by strategies such as periodic reversal of the direction of circulation of the nutrient medium, which significantly improves the culture productivity.

The major advantages of packed-cell over suspension systems for cell culture are that they are more amenable to the use of very low-protein or protein-free media, the cells not being subject to the stress of agitation to keep them in suspension, and that the cell product can accumulate to very high concentrations in the medium around the cells. Both of these features help to make downstream purification of the cell product easier. Problems arise however because, within the cell mass, there will be constant turnover with cells dying and being replaced. This process will release considerable quantities of cell debris, including DNA and intracellular proteases, into the culture supernatant, again reaching high concentrations and presenting problems for product purification and stability.

Suspension culture systems may use either a mechanical agitator or some sort of fluidized bed to mix the cells in the nutrient medium. The stirred tank has the advantage that it is derived directly from the well-established technology developed for bacterial and yeast fermentations and it is well understood. Fluidized bed systems include the air-lift bioreactors that are widely used for monoclonal antibody production. These have the advantage that without a mechanical agitator they are much more simple in their basic operation than are stirred tanks. However air-lifts require addition of antifoams to control foam generation and damage to the cells and their products at the culture surface where the gas leaves the culture medium. Fluidized bed systems using medium recirculation to suspend the cells have the problem that it becomes necessary to encapsulate the cells to retain them within the culture vessel and this introduces a major complication into the preparation of the culture inoculum.

It is now clear that culture conditions can have a substantial effect on the secondary modification of proteins produced by cells *in vitro*. This is particularly marked in the case of glycosylation and it has been shown that this in turn can affect the antigenicity of the protein. This leads on to a general advantage of continuous suspension cultures, that the cells are maintained in a steady state throughout the production process and will produce a more homogeneous product than if the cells are subject to varying conditions whether they arise from gradients within the culture or changes during the culture and the same argument may be expected to apply to products from transgenic animals.

ANIMAL-CELL CULTURE MEDIA

A major problem with the production of recombinant proteins from animal cells is the complexity of the nutrient medium that they require. Typically this medium consists of a number of defined components including at least amino acids, carbohydrates, vitamins and salts, which has traditionally been supplemented by a preparation of macromolecular components, especially proteins, usually in the form of serum from the blood of one of the species of mammal. The serum added to animal-cell culture medium has several functions including cell-growth promotion and cell and product protection from both mechanical and enzymic, especially proteolytic, damage. The main advantages of using serum are that a single reagent, particularly in the form of foetal calf serum, can be used as the medium supplement for a wide range of cell types, it is often very potent in its effect on the cells and can be stored easily for long periods in normal laboratory freezers. The disadvantages of serum include its high protein content (which is poorly defined and much of which is redundant and merely complicates or even interferes with purification of the cell product), it can be a source of infectious contamination of the cell lines, it shows substantial batch-to-batch variation in its cell-culture properties and its availability depends to a large extent on the activity of the meat market which results in cycles of glut and famine. Detailed studies of cell's requirements for growth *in vitro*, prompted by these problems with the serum supplement, have led to development of nutrient media that are either supplemented with purified proteins or with which there is no requirement for a protein supplement at all. However, the more severe the conditions under which the cells are to be cultured, as in stirred tanks, the more complex the formulation of these media has to be. It is, for instance, generally necessary to include a complex lipid supplement, and this results in many serum- or protein-free media being very expensive. These media are also less versatile than serum in that a given formulation can only be used with a restricted range of cell lines, they do not provide protection to the product unless specific enzyme inhibitors are added and there are reports that cell lines are often less stable and less productive in these media than they are in serum supplemented medium. The advantages of serum- or protein-free media are that a very high specific activity of product can be obtained in the culture supernatant, the product accounting for up to 80% of the total protein, thus considerably reducing the problems of downstream purification, the medium composition can be exactly reproduced from batch to batch and there is no danger of introducing infectious contamination.

An option that avoids many of the problems associated with the use of either whole serum or of serum- or protein-free media is to extract subfractions of serum or plasma such that they can be used as cell-culture medium supplements. This has been achieved by reworking Cohn Fraction IV, which is produced as a by-product of routine human plasma fractionation to produce therapeutic blood products and which is otherwise discarded. This product (CMS IV-1) has the advantages of containing much less protein than whole serum but it retains much of the latter's versatility and potency in promoting cell growth, of enhancing productivity and of maintaining cell-line stability. CMS IV-1 contains significant quantities of protease inhibitors which protect the product from degradation during the culture process and it is able to tolerate pasteurization at +60°C for 10 h which has been shown to be very virucidal and effectively removes the risk of introducing infectious contamination by this route. CMS IV-1 is prepared from a product of a validated fractionation process operated under conditions of current pharmaceutical Good Manufacturing Practice and of which the feedstock is plasma derived from the blood of carefully selected donors. Thus CMS IV-1 has less batch-to-batch variation than foetal calf serum and the supply is more dependable and predictable. The main disadvantage of CMS IV-1 is that it is still a complex, undefined mixture of proteins, some of which are still redundant. Some, such as the small amount of residual immunoglobulin, may complicate purification of particular cell products, and the essential active components that promote cell growth have not yet been identified and are almost certainly not present at ideal concentrations.

QUALITY ASSURANCE

To produce a therapeutic protein reproducibly and reliably it is necessary to have a validated process for which the starting materials can be demonstrated to be the same from batch to batch. For an animal-cell culture process, this can be achieved for the nutrient medium by biochemical analysis but for the cells themselves it is necessary to characterize the line and to establish their pedigree. This is done by selecting a clone grown originally from a single cell, selection being on the basis of having optimum culture characteristics in terms of productivity and growth rate and it is then necessary to demonstrate that the cell line is stable for the duration of the cell-culture process. To ensure that every batch of product is produced with identical feedstock it is necessary to freeze (in liquid nitrogen) a number of vials containing cells from the same culture. This collection of frozen vials constitutes a cell bank and by thus ensuring that the cell line does not degenerate through emergence of variants, which would happen if the cells were maintained in culture, the integrity of the production process is assured.

The first cell bank to be produced is the *master cell bank* and while this consists of cells frozen down as soon as possible after the last cloning, it should none the less also be as large as is practicable and if possible should be large enough to last the entire production life of the product. The cells in the master cell bank are characterized as thoroughly as possible with regard to both the cells themselves and the protein product. Thus the features of the cells' genotypes and phenotypes should be established and enough of the protein's biochemical properties to enable it to be unambiguously identified or to reveal whether or not it has been changed during the manufacturing processes to which it is subject. The cells also have to be thoroughly screened to try to ensure that they do not harbour any contaminating organisms such as mycoplasma or viruses.

The next step is to prepare a *manufacturer's working cell bank* by expanding one of the vials from the master cell bank. This again should be as large as is practicable and the cells and their product must be characterized to demonstrate that they are identical with those in the master cell bank. A fresh vial from the manufacturer's working cell bank is used to start each culture from which product is to be recovered for use, thus ensuring that every production culture starts from an inoculum having exactly the same characteristics as all the others.

It is particularly important in the case of cultures that are extended in any way, whether by fed-batch, continuous or perfusion, that the cells and their product are tested again after being in culture for at least as long, and preferably significantly longer, than they would be during the manufacturing process. This is done by keeping cells from the working cell bank in culture for a predetermined period and then freezing them down in an *extended culture cell bank*. This bank of cells is then examined by all the criteria used to characterize the master cell bank to establish whether or not the culture has degenerated through the emergence of non-producing cells or cells producing a protein that is different from that produced by the original cell clone. The extended culture cell bank is also screened for infectious contaminants in the same way as the master cell bank in case a very low level contaminant was missed in the original screening but has proliferated sufficiently in culture to be detected.

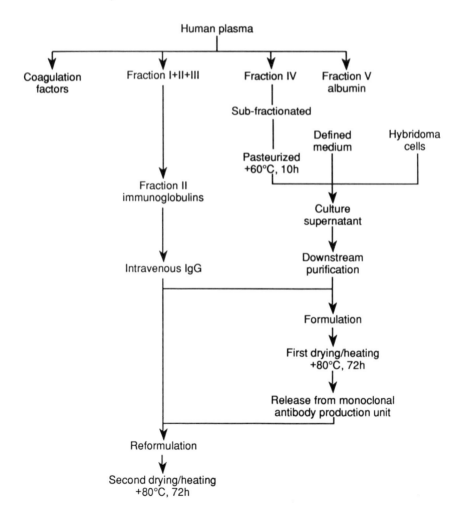

Fig. 4.5. Process outline: integration of plasma fractionation and monoclonal antibody production

INTEGRATION WITH EXISTING MANUFACTURING OPERATIONS

While it is obviously possible, and in some respects desirable, to establish manufacturing units for the production of therapeutic proteins using recombinant DNA or hybridoma technology in a facility dedicated to this process, there are also advantages to be gained from associating it with a pre-existing centre, such as a plasma fractionation plant, producing similar products. The benefits of such an association arise from the many features of the plant which can be used by the cell-culture development and which reduce the burden of overhead costs during the early stages of the programme, and from the existence of a Quality Assurance system which ensures that the emerging technology develops in compliance with current pharmaceutical Good Manufacturing Practice. A model for such an association for the production of a therapeutic monoclonal antibody has been developed at the Protein Fractionation Centre of the Scottish National Blood Transfusion Service in Edinburgh. In this case, hybridoma cells are cultured in medium supplemented with human protein derived from Cohn Fraction IV-1 and the final antibody product is formulated in normal human immune globulin for intravenous administration (Figure 4.5). As mentioned above, this programme benefits from the manufacturing facilities and Quality Assurance system established for the plasma fractionation process as well as transforming a discarded by-product of that process into a valuable feedstock and is also able to use the mechanisms established for organization of clinical evaluation of the normal human plasma products.

FURTHER READING

Ausebel, F.M. *et al* (Eds) (1987) *Current Protocols in Molecular Biology*, Vols 1 and 2. Greene Publishing Associates/Wiley-Interscience, New York. (Regularly updated with supplements.)

Bliem, R. (1988) Aspects of process development in animal cell technology. *Pharmaceutical Engineering*, 8(6), 15–19.

Darnell, J., Lodish, H. and Baltimore, D. (Eds) (1990) *Molecular Cell Biology*, 2nd edn. Scientific American Books, San Francisco.

EEC Guidelines on Medicinal Products Derived from Modern Biotechnological Processes (1989) *Journal of Biological Standardization*, 17, 201–231.

Hames, B.D. and Glover, D.M. (Eds) (1988) *Transcription and Splicing*. IRL Press.

Spier, R.E. and Griffiths, J.B. (Eds) (1990) *Animal Cell Biotechnology*, Vols 1–5. Academic Press, London.

Watson, J.D., Hopkins, N.H., Roberts, J.W., Steitz, J.A. and Weiner, A.M. (Eds) (1987) *Molecular Biology of the Gene*, 4th edn., Vols 1 and 2. Benjamin/Cummings, Menlo Park, CA.

5 New Approaches to Product Isolation

T. BURNOUF

INTRODUCTION

For many years, plasma fractionation technology has been limited to the isolation of albumin, immunoglobulin G (IgG), and clotting factors by precipitation methods (see Chapter 3). The low selectivity of precipitation methods in general have, however, been a drawback to improving the purification factor of labile plasma proteins as well as to isolating 'new' plasma proteins with potential clinical interest. Today, plasma fractionators must turn to new purification technology. This drive towards innovation is dictated for several reasons:

- Over the years, medical research has discovered links between specific diseases and congenital or acquired plasma protein deficiency, thus pointing out the need for new plasma derivatives to be used for substitutive therapy.
- The viral risk associated with crude plasma fractions has been recognized, thus requiring the treatment of patients by virus-safe, purified plasma products.
- Some plasma preparations, because of their overload in protein contaminants, may have deleterious immunological effects in patients.
- The limited supply of human plasma makes the production of new plasma derivatives mandatory to permit selective hemotherapy whenever possible.
- Economical considerations necessitate lowering the present cost of plasma fractionation technology through an improved efficiency of the purification methods and an increased diversity of products isolated from plasma.
- Countries, especially those in the less developed world, may wish to develop their own plasma fractionation industry using new, possibly less costly and more flexible purification procedures.

In parallel to the need seen in the improvement of plasma fractionation technology, the development of genetic engineering and cell-fusion technology

Plasma and Recombinant Blood Products in Medical Therapy
Edited by C.V. Prowse.   Published 1992 by John Wiley & Sons Ltd

has opened the way to an alternative source of plasma proteins. Both fields require the successful implementation of efficient purification methods. Downstream processing from both plasma and synthetic sources plays a central role in the therapeutic efficiency and safety of such protein-based therapeutics; it characterizes the product in a precise succession of purification steps that influences purity, viral safety and potential antigenicity.

Present purification methodologies involve the use of open-column liquid chromatography which has already become a pre-eminent technique for isolating and recovering several plasma proteins, providing both good yield and good purity. This technique is a major aspect of consideration in plasma fractionation and biotechnological production.

Here the parameters and features attached to the choice of chromatography in plasma protein purification are presented. Major applications are also described.

CHROMATOGRAPHIC MATRICES

When it comes to choosing a chromatographic system, careful consideration should be given to the selection of the matrix since its properties and chemical nature greatly influence the overall performance and adaptability of the procedure to large-scale fractionation.

PROPERTIES

A chromatographic gel or support is a matrix on which active sites may be bound. Although the matrix should not interact with the plasma proteins or buffer components, its type may influence the design of a protein purification scheme.

Ideally a matrix for large-scale application should have the following properties:

Rigidity. This allows high flow rate without gel deformation and plugging. Rigidity is important when column adsorption of several hundreds of litres of a plasma fraction must be achieved.

Bead uniformity. Uniformity in size and shape improves gel performance and resolution.

Chemical and biological stability. To avoid any pyrogenic substances, supports must be resistant to cleansing agents such as sodium hydroxide or acid solutions. Resistance to autoclaving is an advantage to comply with Good Manufacturing Practices, for example, viral or bacterial decontamination. The beads should be chemically and biologically inert towards proteins and buffer components to avoid the leaching of harmful materials in the therapeutic fractions, and to avoid biochemical modifications, such as the activation of clotting factors. This is of special importance for plasma protein concentrates injected under large infusion volumes and/or long-term treatment.

Low non-specific interaction. Non-specific interaction, in addition to modifying the chemistry of a matrix, may decrease column performance and limit column life-time.

Porous network. Porosity is relevant in adsorption chromatography of plasma proteins because they differ very much in size. Molecular weights of plasma proteins range from ca. 30000 daltons to over 20 million daltons. Large-pore supports allow macromolecules access to active sites while minimizing gel filtration effect.

Constancy. Characteristics of the matrix from batch to batch and from cycle to cycle must be constant to permit reproducible separations and avoid non-specific interactions leading to uncontrolled binding. This latter point is important in terms of the chromatographic behaviour of viruses particularly for products whose virus safety is dependent upon the purification process.

CHOICE

The following matrices have been used in the purification of plasma proteins:

Cellulose. Cellulose is a linear polymer of β1,4-linked D-glucose units with occasional 1,6-bonds and was among the first media to be used in plasma protein fractionation. The usual forms have an irregular fibrous structure and are difficult to pack in columns. Their pore size is small and non-specific adsorption may occur. DEAE-derivatized cellulose still has a limited use as an ion exchanger in the isolation of crude fractions such as the prothrombin complex (PCC). Nevertheless, cellulose-based media tend to be restricted to once-off disposable application to achieve preliminary purification from crude protein fractions prior to high-resolution purification.

Agarose. Agarose is a linear, galactose-containing colloid commonly used in plasma fractionation chromatographic processes, especially for ion exchange and affinity. Major brands used in plasma fractionation are Sepharose (Pharmacia), Ultrogel A (IBF) and Biogel A (Bio-Rad). The advantages include high gel strength, biological inertness, and limited non-specific adsorption. Cross-linked agarose (Sepharose CL) has improved flow characteristics, increased stability to chaotropic agents and resistance to cleansing procedures with sodium hydroxide, a common cleansing agent in the plasma fractionation industry. In contrast, organic solvents (such as ethanol) should have restricted use since they may induce irreversible changes in the gel structure. Agarose-based ion exchangers probably represent the most popular matrix in the large-scale purification of many plasma proteins including albumin, Factor VIII (FVIII), Factor IX (FIX) and various protease inhibitors.

Dextran. Dextran is an α-1,6-linked glucose polymer. The cross-linked forms (Sephadex, Pharmacia) are often used in plasma derivative production, especially as gel filtration and ion-exchange media. Cross-linked dextrans have low non-specific binding and are resistant to dilute sodium hydroxide and hydrochloric acid solutions. Sephadex can be reversibly swollen from the dried state with no detectable influence on the chromatographic proper-ties. The swollen Sephadex can be cleansed by autoclaving with no signifi-cant changes in its properties. Sephadex G-25, one of the highly cross-linked forms, has found a specific use for the desalting of plasma protein fractions prior to a chromatographic step and/or whenever desalting by gel filtration induces less alteration to proteins than does ultrafiltration. DEAE-Sephadex A-50 is an anion exchanger which has often replaced DEAE-cellulose for the isolation of PCC. It is also now being used as a preliminary concentration and crude purification step in the production of highly-purified FIX, prior to more selective anion-exchange steps.

Polyacrylamide and polyacrylamide-based media. Polyacrylamide is composed of a hydrocarbon backbone with carboxyamide side-chains. It is used as such (Bio-gel P) or combined with agarose (Ultrogel AcA) or with dextran (Sephacryl, Pharmacia). Polyacrylamide gels are stable from pH 1 to 10, which prohibits severe cleansing with sodium hydroxide. Some advantages are its biological inertness and its resistance to attack from microorganisms, but autoclaving is not possible. It is not frequently used in plasma fractiona-tion, possibly because acrylamide compressibility and resistance to flow makes large-scale column chromatography unsatisfactory.

Polyacrylamide-agarose beds are rigid and thus more adapted to industrial separations. They include both gel-filtration media and affinity media. The structure of the various types of Ultrogel-AcA is based on a three-dimensional network of polyacrylamide enclosing an agarose gel. The porosity of the gel depends on the content of polyacrylamide.

Polyacrylamide-dextran beds of different porosities have found their niche in plasma fractionation. For example, Sephacryl S-200 and Sephacryl S-200 HR are used as the final purification step of both chromatographically-purified albumin and α_1-antitrypsin (AAT) to remove high-molecular-weight (HMW) contaminants.

Trisacryl. Trisacryl (IBF), a synthetic medium, is a polymer of *N*-acryloyl-2-amino-2-hydroxymethyl-1,3-propanediol. Advantages include high hydrophilicity, non-biodegradability, thermostability and resistance to autoclaving and detergents. DEAE-Trisacryl AR has an improved stability to basic pH, making cleansing with sodium hydroxide possible. The use of such matrices has been reported for gel filtration, ion exchange, and affinity chromatography of plasma proteins. One major application is the purification of IgG.

Eupergit. Eupergit (Röhm Pharma) is an oxirane acrylic chromatographic support made by the copolymerization of methacrylamide, methylene-bis (methacrylamide), and allyl-glycidyl ether. Beads are spherical and have a mean diameter of 140–180 μm. The macroporous structure (pore diameter 0.1–3 μm), good mechanical stability and resistance to flow-rate make it well adapted to large-scale column chromatography. This matrix is stable from pH 1 to 12 for several hours at room temperature. Heparin-Eupergit has been reported as suitable for the purification of antithrombin III (ATIII) from human plasma.

Fractogel. Fractogel TSK (Toya-Soda, Merck) is a synthetic macroporous vinyl polymer matrix obtained by the copolymerization of oligoethyleneglycol, glycidylmethacrylate and pentaerythroldimethacrylate. Beads are spherical with narrow particle size distribution. The high mechanical stability enables high elution rate. Resistance to pH 1–14, along with its chemical stability and compatibility with chaotropic agents and organic solvents, facilitates cleaning procedures. Autoclaving is possible. Fractogel-based chromatographic gels are available for gel filtration, ion exchange, hydrophobic interaction and affinity chromatography. One important application is in the purification of a new generation of high-purity FVIII, and von Willebrand factor (vWF) concentrates.

Controlled-pore glass (CPG). CPG (Corning) is obtained by heating selected borosilicate glasses to 500–800°C for prolonged periods of time. Upon heat treatment, the glass mixture separates into borate- and silica-rich phases: the borate phase, then dissolved by acid, is coated to block the silanol groups and thus limit its ionic character. CPG has been used in the manufacturing of intermediate-purity FVIII concentrate.

CHROMATOGRAPHIC METHODS IN PLASMA FRACTIONATION

Chromatography has gained importance in plasma fractionation because it separates and isolates biologically active molecules without disrupting their biological features. Providing selectivity, efficiency and versatility, it is well adapted to the specific objective of plasma fractionation because simultaneous

Table 5.1 Examples of the use of chromatography in the purification of plasma-derived products used in clinics

Name	Principles
Albumin	IEC, SEC
IgG	IEC
Clotting factors	
FVIII	IEC, SEC, mAb affinity
vWF	IEC, affinity (dextran sulphate)
FIX	IEC, mAb
FII, FVII, FX	IEC
Protein C	IEC, mAb affinity
Fibrinogen	IEC, affinity (heparin)
Protease inhibitors	
ATIII	IEC, affinity (heparin)
AAT (α_1PI)	IEC, SEC
C1-inhibitor	IEC
Fibronectin	Affinity (gelatin, heparin)
Plasminogen	Affinity (lysine)

recovery of a number of therapeutic proteins can be achieved. Only a few chromatographic techniques have found their niche in industrial plants; those in use have been shown to be an effective tool in the downstream processing of plasma proteins.

Plasma protein chromatographic purification often relies on three different purification principles: ion exchange, biospecific conventional affinity and size exclusion. Monoclonal antibody affinity has recently been introduced to purify some clotting factors. Hydrophobic interaction is still rarely used. Procedures generally combine various chromatographic principles to ensure a good level of purity of the targeted protein (Table 5.1).

CHROMATOGRAPHIC PRINCIPLES

Ion-exchange chromatography

The amino acid side chains of plasma proteins carry ionic charges that result in adsorption to suitably charged ion exchangers. The separation mechanism depends on the ionic interaction between charged molecules on the stationary phase in the mobile phase and ionic protein species. The net charge of proteins are pH dependent, thus influencing their binding capacity to ion exchangers. At a pH below its isoelectric point, or pI, a protein has a positive net charge (due to protonization of amino acid side chains) and, above its pI, a negative net charge, permitting binding to negatively and positively charged ion exchangers, respectively.

Ion exchangers can be classified into two types: anionic when carrying positive charges, cationic when carrying negative charges. Anionic exchangers are considered as weak when they are derived from a weak base (e.g. diethylaminoethyl, DEAE) or strong when derived from a strong acid (quaternary aminoethyl, QAE). Similarly, weak (carboxymethyl, CM) and strong (sulphopropyl, SP) cationic exchangers are distinguished. A major difference between those two types is that strong ion exchangers retain their charge over a pH range broader than that of weak ion exchangers. This phenomenon influences the separation parameters since variations in buffer pH may affect the net charge of both protein and weak ion exchangers. For example, an increase in pH may increase the net negative charge of the protein (as more amino acid side chains lose protons) while, at the same time, lowering the positive charge of a weak anion exchanger and thus decreasing the strength of adsorption.

Ion-exchange chromatography (IEC) is well adapted to the separation of proteins from complex plasma mixtures. It separates into groups those proteins bearing comparable net charges. Since plasma proteins do not exhibit the same degree or type of interaction with the ion exchanger, the strength of adsorption to the charged groups will differ, thus permitting differential elution. IEC can be considered as being an almost ideal plasma protein separation technique at any part of the fractionation process, but is especially helpful at the beginning of a purification scheme.

The elution of proteins can be obtained by changing either the pH of the chromatographic buffer or its ionic strength, by adding counter ions (e.g. sodium chloride, acetate, or phosphate) that compete with bound proteins for the charged groups of the solid phase. Whereas precise pH variations are difficult to achieve, ionic strength variations can readily be made to achieve highly selective elutions. In most cases, the salt concentration is changed in a stepwise manner to elute proteins.

The most usual form of ion exchange is anionic since at neutral pH many plasma proteins, which have a pI between 4.5 and 6.5, carry a negative net charge. Anion exchangers are frequently used to bind and concentrate the target protein(s). A significant exception to this rule is IgG which, especially for subclasses 1, 2 and 3, is one of the more basic plasma protein classes: when chromatographed on a weak anion exchanger at neutral pH, an essentially pure IgG fraction can be recovered in the unbound fraction. This characteristic has brought about a new and interesting application of anion exchangers in the purification of plasma proteins obtained by immunoaffinity: the elimination or reduction of potential contamination with murine monoclonal antibodies (mAb).

To date, cation exchangers have been relatively under-exploited in plasma protein purification. They can be of significant interest in the removal of protein contaminants provided the buffer conditions, especially pH, are well selected to segregate them from the target protein. Binding on cation exchangers at slightly acid pH may also be of some interest in the purification and concentration of IgG.

For most plasma proteins, it is unlikely that a single IEC step could have a very high degree of specificity. The general nature of the adsorption principle (electrostatic interaction) leads to similar interactions for a variety of different plasma proteins and, consequently, to the co-elution of biochemically related molecules. One ion-exchange step can be expected to achieve an average purification of $\leq$ 10-fold, but the combination of several ion exchangers may permit a significant degree of purification. An example is the 10000-fold purification of FIX obtained by the chromatography of plasma cryosupernatant successively on DEAE-Sephadex A-50, DEAE-Sepharose CL-6B fast-flow and heparin-Sepharose.

Affinity chromatography

The most important development in chromatography pertaining to plasma protein purification is the introduction of affinity chromatography. This mode of separation involves an immobilized ligand, covalently attached to the stationary phase, which effects a highly specific biological interaction with a given protein. The degree of selectivity is highly dependent on the capacity of the ligand to interact with the target protein and not with other ones. The degree of interaction between ligand and protein should not be too high, however, to avoid harsh conditions of desorption that would irreversibly alter functionality. Elution is performed usually by stepwise increase of the salt concentration or by specific eluants. Chromatographic matrices should be selected to allow the best immobilization of the ligand, good stability and suitable performance. Although ligands may be of very different nature (amino acids, polysaccharides, proteins, dyes, chelated metals, lectins, enzyme inhibitors) their actual use in large-scale purification of therapeutic plasma proteins has so far been limited to those demonstrated to be compatible with the therapeutic use of the target protein(s). For example, immobilized heparin has been described in the production of concentrates of ATIII and fibrinogen, lysine and gelatin in that of fibrinogen and fibronectin, respectively. Mouse mAb have recently been used to isolate plasma FVIII and FIX.

At least in theory, this technique combines simplicity and specificity. However, it has a limited interest in the early stages of plasma fractionation, and is best used as the last step of the purification process. Applying affinity chromatography early in a fractionation process could indeed be inconvenient since the performance of the gel may be impaired due to non-specific binding, and the presence of proteolytic enzymes may affect the ligand structure.

Size-exclusion chromatography

Size-exclusion chromatography (SEC) separates, under isocratic conditions, proteins according to their size (or hydrodynamic volume) on an inert, macroporous, stationary support with controlled pore sizes. SEC is certainly the most predictable chromatographic separation method as long as it is not run in conditions of extreme ionic strength which favour interferences between proteins and the support. Since separations in plasma fractionation are often carried out under near-physiological conditions, such interferences can be regarded as rare.

Optimal separation in SEC requires small, concentrated sample volume as compared to column size along with relatively low flow rates. SEC is not convenient for early separation steps of plasma proteins but may be advantageous for final purification of reasonably pure solutions. SEC can also be used to desalt a fraction, to equilibrate a protein solution in a new buffer system adapted to downstream processing (e.g. ion exchange or affinity), or to remove low-molecular-weight reagents (such as stabilizers used during viral inactivation).

Examples of SEC in plasma fractionation include the final purification step of AAT and albumin on Sephacryl S-200. Desalting by SEC has been described for ATIII to remove the stabilizer used during pasteurization, for IgG to equilibrate the protein solution to correct buffer conditions prior to chromatographic purification, and for albumin to remove the ethanol used during the Cohn fractionation process.

Hydrophobic interaction

Hydrophobic interaction chromatography (HIC) separates on the basis of interactions between exposed non-polar amino acid residues on the protein surface and the hydrophobic groups of the adsorbent. Ligands are usually hydrocarbonaceous entities (butyl, pentyl, octyl, phenyl). Adsorption of proteins occurs under high ionic strength conditions and elution is performed by decreasing salt concentrations. In contrast to reversed-phase chromatography, HIC uses bonded stationary phase with ligands of relatively low density or hydrophobicity and, consequently, organic solvents are not required to achieve elution, thereby allowing preparative purification and a good recovery of biological activity. Sometimes, however, strong interactions between certain proteins and these gels can make it difficult to obtain high recovery rates due to incomplete desorption or to a loss in activity resulting from the use of stronger eluants.

In principle, HIC could be used at any step of a fractionation procedure but would be particularly beneficial following a precipitation step under high salt concentration. There are only limited examples of the use of HIC in plasma protein fractionation. An approach has been made to use octanohydrazide-Sepharose to bind and eliminate lipid-enveloped viruses from PCC.

PURIFICATION STRATEGY AND CONSTRAINTS

Objectives

The objective of process selection in most biotechnological areas is to define the shortest and most realistic scheme to obtain a highly purified product with maximum yield and minimized cost. This scheme should be well adapted to conditions where only a single protein is to be purified from a given source. However, purification strategy in plasma fractionation is regulated by specific rules:

- In already-established fractionation plants, chromatography is a relatively new approach to isolate plasma proteins: consequently it must be introduced in a manner compatible to the pre-existing bulk ethanol fractionation process. Modifications to an established process could disqualify the pharmacological and clinical data of existing products.
- Purification processes must ensure compatible and parallel production of the many plasma protein fractions that have clinical use. Thus, the objective is not necessarily to obtain the highest possible recovery for all therapeutic proteins: rather, it is to design a complex fractionation process that ensures the best possible compatibility in the purification of a number of proteins to procure all the plasma derivatives needed in a given area. This may lead to the design of a production process which is efficient for a protein known to be in high demand clinically, at the relative expense of by-products with minor clinical importance.

General design of process

The separation of plasma derivatives from crude plasma fractions is best based on multiple-step procedures that ensure a satisfactory degree of purity to the main target proteins while permitting recovery of by-product fractions with potential therapeutic interest.

The first chromatographic separation step must have a selectivity high enough to remove most of the water and the bulk proteins not sharing biochemical properties with the protein(s) of interest. Selectivity during the first purification, however, does not need to be high. Indeed, the objective is to get a concentrated, semi-purified fraction that facilitates subsequent handling of the product, saving in further processing time, and possible storage under an appropriate form. Integrated to the existing ethanol fractionation process, the first chromatographic step should then be designed so that the protein(s) looked upon is (are) bound on the chromatographic material in conditions where the bulk proteins are found in the unbound fractions and can be easily recovered for further processing. Such a design may also remove plasma-borne proteolytic enzymes that could impair

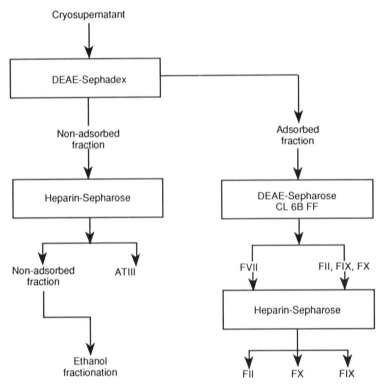

Fig. 5.1. Outline of the series of anion exchange and affinity chromatographic steps used in the purification of FVII, FIX and ATIII (CRTS, Lille)

further purification of labile protein. Chromatography can be used to purify plasma proteins from essentially any existing plasma fraction.

Examples

Factor IX

The isolation of FIX presents an example of the use of a combination of several IEC steps (Figure 5.1). A crude extraction of FIX is first carried out by batch adsorption of cryosupernatant on DEAE-Sephadex A50 so as to isolate PCC. The bound fraction, containing FIX, is eluted and further purified by a more efficient anion exchanger (DEAE-Sepharose CL-6B fast-flow) to segregate major proteins of the PCC. The mixture is injected onto a column equilibrated in a buffer at a pH slightly lower than the pI of most of the proteins in the mixture. Various increases in the ionic strength elute fractions enriched in various proteins such as FVII and FIX. In this chromatographic step, the increase in the purity of FIX is about threefold and no clear separation from FII and FX occurs, but proteins or zymogens which could interfere with the purification of FIX are removed. Separation of FIX from FII and FX is carried out by a highly selective chromatographic step using heparin-bound agarose, these two proteins having a lower binding capacity to heparin than does FIX. The resulting FIX has a specific activity on the order of 100 IU/mg and is purified over 30-fold by this heparin chromatographic step. The overall purification factor from plasma is about 10 000-fold.

This process illustrates how a traditional adsorption step of human plasma can be exploited to make, through a series of chromatographic steps of increasing selectivity, a new, high-purity clotting factor fraction, along with other potentially new plasma derivatives, without having an impact on the industrial ethanol fractionation process.

Antithrombin III (ATIII)

An example of the combination of IEC and affinity chromatography can be found in the procedure employed to purify ATIII (Figure 5.1), a potent protease inhibitor also called heparin cofactor. ATIII can be produced by chromatography of DEAE Sephadex-adsorbed cryosupernatant on insoluble heparin, in conditions having minimal influence on the bulk fractionation process. Albumin and IgG are found in the non-adsorbed fraction and can be processed by cold ethanol fractionation. A washing step at increased ionic strength elutes a fraction which contains contaminants to be discarded. ATIII is eluted by further increasing the salt concentration of the buffer.

The use of fraction IV-1 as a starting material has also been described; there is even less interference with the main fractionation process because the starting material is an unused by-product of routine plasma fractionation. However, the recovery is much reduced due to a loss in fractions II + III, incomplete precipitation and altered state of ATIII in fraction IV-1, and the limited solubility of this latter fraction.

Affinity chromatography, in addition to being an elegant and efficient purification means, may also have advantages in segregating active and inactive forms of plasma proteins. For example, heparin-agarose-purified ATIII is subjected to viral inactivation by heat treatment at 60°C for 10 h in the liquid state. This virus inactivation treatment induces some degree of denaturation which is apparent from the loss in the capacity of some of the ATIII to bind heparin. It has been shown that heparin-agarose adsorption of pasteurized ATIII is capable of selectively adsorbing and separating the unaltered form from the altered forms. This property is presently used in some fractionation plants to prepare fully active, virus-inactivated ATIII concentrate.

α_1-Antitrypsin

Purification of AAT from human plasma represents an example of a combined use of IEC and SEC (Figure 5.2). In the process described by the CRTS

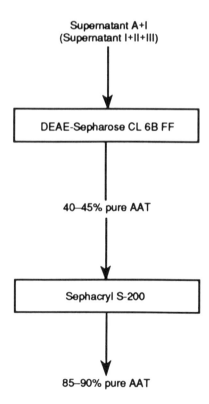

Fig. 5.2. Example of the combination of IEC and SEC in the purification of AAT (CRTS, Lille)

of Lille, supernatant II + III is first chromatographed on DEAE-Sepharose CL 6B fast-flow to ensure the pre-purification of AAT. The column is equilibrated in a neutral buffer under conditions which remove any IgG still present in the starting material. A washing step at lower pH elutes a fraction containing > 90% pure transferrin. Albumin is recovered by lowering the pH of the buffer (pH 4.5) below its pI where it has an overall positive charge. The ionic strength of this buffer is low enough to prohibit elution of AAT. The next step at increased pH and ionic strength elutes a pre-purified AAT fraction. The purity of the product at this stage of the procedure is between 40 and 45%. Subsequent SEC of the concentrated and dialyzed fraction on Sephacryl S-200 eliminates protein contaminants. The resulting purity of the product is between 85 and 90%. No significant problems of reproducibility and efficiency have been encountered when applying this SEC step on a large scale.

Factor VIII and von Willebrand Factor (vWF)

Purification by conventional adsorption chromatography The possibility of applying adsorption chromatography to the large-scale manufacture of FVIII
and vWF concentrates is new, in spite of many attempts which have been
made in the past using resins such as ECTEOLA or Amino-hexyl agarose.
Results were unsatisfactory due to low chromatographic yields and the
instability of FVIII. Consequently, until the last few years, cryoprecipitate, or

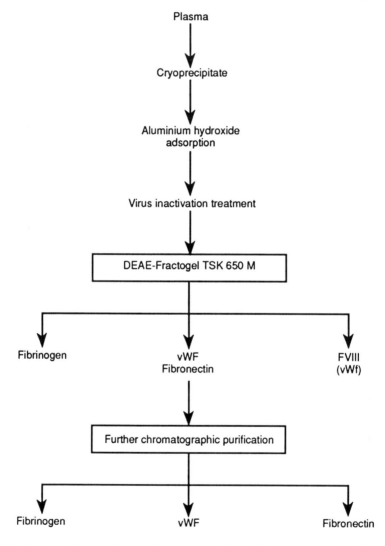

Fig. 5.3. Use of anion exchange chromatography in the course of purification of
FVIII, vWF, fibrinogen and fibronectin from cryoprecipitate (CRTS-Lille)

concentrates obtained by crude precipitation steps from cryoprecipitate, have been the sole sources for the treatment of haemophilia A and von Willebrand patients.

The chromatographic procedure of the CRTS of Lille to produce highly purified FVIII and vWF concentrates is based on the separation and selectivity afforded by DEAE-Fractogel TSK 650M (Figure 5.3). This anion exchanger, among several other commercial resins studied, has been shown to have a high binding capacity for the FVIII/vWF complex and low 'affinity' for most of the protein contaminants of the cryoprecipitate, especially fibrinogen and IgG. The cryoprecipitate solution is injected onto the resin after aluminium hydroxide adsorption and virus inactivation treatment. Most proteins flow through the gel unretarded: these include fibrinogen, IgG, albumin (which was entrapped in the cryoprecipitate) and some fibronectin. A washing step made at a higher salt content elutes a fraction containing vWF and fibronectin. Finally, a further increase in the ionic strength elutes FVIII, under good conditions for yield and stability. The average purification of FVIII achieved by this chromatographic step is about 200-fold, a purification factor which is remarkable for an ion exchanger and which argues in favour of some 'affinity' interaction playing a role in this separation. The overall purification factor from plasma is over 10000-fold. The specific activity of the final product is about 170 IU FVIII:c/mg.

The recovery of the vWF + fibronectin wash fraction and its further processing by additional chromatographic steps, including DEAE-Fractogel, discriminates between vWF and fibronectin and allows production of a vWF concentrate with a specific activity exceeding 100 U ristocetin cofactor/mg. The content of high-molecular-weight vWF multimers (several million daltons) in this concentrate has been shown to be equivalent to that in plasma: this confirms that the Fractogel chromatographic support has a pore size permitting the retention of very large entities.

Fibrinogen and fibronectin can be recovered from the unbound DEAE-Fractogel chromatographic filtrate and the wash fraction, respectively. Several approaches can be used to purify fibrinogen, including binding it on immobilized heparin in order to remove the IgG and the albumin that contaminate the unbound DEAE Fractogel filtrate. Similarly, fibronectin can be purified by affinity chromatography on gelatin-bound chromatographic supports.

This chromatographic procedure can be easily integrated with the classical production method of virus-inactivated, intermediate-purity FVIII, and does not interfere with the production of the other major plasma derivatives, provides highly purified products, and allows simultaneous recovery of the major proteins of the cryoprecipitate, thus favoring the optimal use of human plasma.

Immunopurification technique Immunopurification technology has been developed recently in an attempt to produce 'ultrapure' FVIII concentrates.

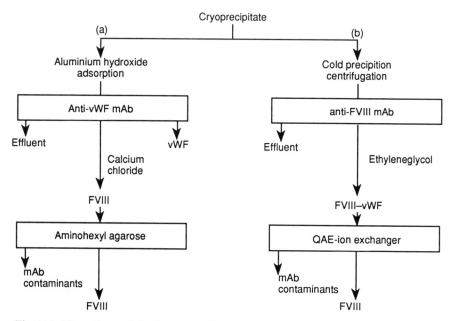

Fig. 5.4. Flow-sheet of the immunoaffinity purification of FVIII using (a) anti-vWF mAb (Monoclate, Armour) and (b) anti-FVIII mAb (Hemophil M, Baxter)

Since most FVIII circulates in plasma as a complex with vWF, this approach consists of using mAb directed against one protein of the complex. Such antibodies possess affinity for a single epitope of the antigen. By binding the antibody to a suitable matrix support, it has become theoretically possible to achieve a highly biospecific purification of FVIII.

In one procedure (used to produce 'Monoclate', from Armour), a mAb directed to vWF is used (Figure 5.4a). The cryoprecipitate is suspended and then subjected to aluminium hydroxide adsorption to remove vitamin-K dependent clotting factors. The adsorbed cryoprecipitate is subsequently applied to an anti-vWF mAb covalently bound to a Sepharose matrix to adsorb the FVIII–vWF complex. Extensive washing of the gel removes the non-adsorbed proteins. FVIII is eluted with calcium-containing solution which dissociates it from the vWF. The vWF remains bound to the antibody and is subsequently dissociated from the antibody by elution with thiocyanate. Further processing of the FVIII fraction includes a concentration step by ultrafiltration and subsequent binding on an aminohexyl agarose column. This last chromatographic step was designed to reduce the level of mAb that had leached from the column, and to provide additional purification of FVIII from protein contaminants.

The other process (used to produce Hemophil M, from Baxter) employs a mouse mAb directed against the FVIII molecule (Figure 5.4b). The cryoprecipitate is first dissolved in water and then subjected to cold precipitation and centrifugation to reduce the level of fibrinogen and fibronectin and to clarify the solution. After virus inactivation, the resulting supernatant is next applied to the anti-FVIII mAb column. Most of the cryoprecipitate proteins flow through the gel unretarded, whereas FVIII is bound. Elution of FVIII is subsequently achieved by applying a solution containing 40% ethyleneglycol to the column. Further purification, mainly to eliminate contaminating mAb, is performed by chromatography on a QAE matrix to which FVIII binds. Under the conditions chosen, the ionic strength in the chromatographic separation was high enough to limit the binding of mAb to the anion exchanger.

Due to their specificity, these two immunopurification methods permit a high degree of purification of FVIII, although its final specific activity is relatively low (about 5 IU/mg) due to the stabilization with albumin. Drawbacks of such procedures, from the plasma fractionator standpoint, are found in the difficulty of combining this purification approach with the recovery of other therapeutic subfractions of the cryoprecipitate and, from the clinician and patient standpoints, in the side effects potentially associated with the residual detectable contamination of mouse mAb.

PURIFICATION OF PROTEINS FROM NON-PLASMA SOURCES

Progress in molecular and cell biology, through recombinant DNA (rDNA) technology and cell fusion, has made the production of synthetic proteins from sources other than plasma possible (see Chapters 4, 6 and 8). Benefits seen from such an approach are (1) the elimination of the risk of transmission of plasma-born viruses and (2) increased availability. In the 1980s, the genes coding many important plasma proteins were cloned and expressed in various cells while hybridoma technology was evaluated for the production of mAb, especially against viral or bacterial agents. Clinical trials of recombinant FVIII and anti-Rhesus mAb to assess their efficiency and safety are in progress.

Downstream processing plays a central role in the efficiency and safety of these new protein-based therapeutics since a number of steps may potentially alter labile proteins. The challenge in the production of 'synthetic proteins' is the design of a mild purification method to avoid the inactivation of biological activity, while providing extreme purity and good yield. Achieving the highest degree of purity of the targeted protein is mandatory. Harmful contaminants to be eliminated include proteins, DNA, or viruses originating from the production system. The difficulties encountered in the purification of recombinant plasma proteins are linked to the production system and to the complexity of the culture medium.

PRODUCTION SYSTEM

Some important parameters are the ability of the host production system to express the protein in a native state and to secrete it or not into the culture medium.

The bacterium *Escherichia coli* is the favourite host of genetic engineers because (1) several vector plasmids can be used, (2) it is well adapted to mass culture in fermenter, and (3) the level of expression is generally high (several grams per litre). Although albumin and AAT have been produced by transformed *E. coli*, it is of limited interest for most plasma protein because post-translational modifications cannot be performed. Proteins are rarely excreted and tend to accumulate in the cytoplasm as aggregates or inclusion bodies, making it necessary to break the cells to recover the protein. The downstream purification process must eliminate cell-membrane components, host proteins, and other potential contaminants, such as endotoxins (which are excreted by *E. coli*).

The yeast *Saccharomyces cerevisiae* has a fairly high expression level (a few hundred milligrams per litre) and is capable of post-translational modifications (limited proteolysis and basic glycosylation). Although the production and secretion of human serum albumin at > 1 g/litre has been described, protein often accumulates in the cytoplasm and must be extracted after destruction of the cell. Consequently, the purification process must be designed to eliminate cell components.

Mammalian cells are often chosen for the production of human plasma proteins since they synthesize highly complex molecules with molecular weights exceeding 50 kDa and perform complex post-translational processing (such as γ-carboxylation and glycosylation). The purification process is facilitated as proteins are generally secreted but the expression level remains much lower than that afforded by *E. coli* and *S. cerevisiae*.

Other production systems, developed more recently, include bacteria (*Bacillus*), moulds (*Streptomyces, Aspergillus*), yeasts (*Pichia pastoris, Kluyveromyces lactis*) and baculovirus transformed-insect cells (*Spodoptera frugiperda*). Each of these systems carries its own purification problem but, basically, the separation scheme must follow that used for other systems, as the purity of the final product is a major consideration. A recent approach is the use of transgenic animals. For instance, genetically modified sheep can express human FIX or AAT in the mammary gland, secreting these proteins in the milk. Rabbits were also transformed to synthesize AAT in the blood. The expression of proteins in milk is a good approach since collection of the raw material is easy and purification is less complicated than from blood. Plants transformed by *Agrobacterium tumefasciens* have recently produced plasma proteins. Examples include mouse IgG in tobacco and human serum albumin in potatoes. The purification scheme is highly dependent upon the secreting organ or system (e.g. cell culture, leaf, seed or grain) which may contain specific proteolytic enzymes potentially affecting the recovery of the targeted protein.

INFLUENCE OF CULTURE MEDIUM AND CONDITIONS

Cell culture and purification must be considered as a single process. The choice of a suitable culture medium is important since its composition may interfere with the purification of the cell-secreted protein, especially when the targeted protein is very diluted in the medium. When producing hybridomas, the media should comprise human proteins (such as albumin or transferrin) exclusively, to avoid the contamination problems associated with the use of animal proteins after purification. Further, serum-free media make the purification of biomolecules easier.

CHROMATOGRAPHIC APPROACH

Chromatography may separate proteins of endocellular origin or those secreted by cells into the culture medium. The combination of different chromatographic techniques may achieve a high degree of purification.

IEC is convenient as a first purification step since, after suitable adjustment of pH and ionic strength, it may adsorb the protein of interest, and lead to a more concentrated, partially purified solution. IEC has commonly been applied to the purification of mAb from hybridoma culture supernatants.

HIC is an interesting adsorption step after an ammonium sulphate precipitation performed to concentrate the targeted protein from the culture medium. Chromatographic parameters should be adjusted to avoid drastic conditions which might affect the biological activity.

SEC is helpful any time the components to be separated are very different in size, or when a desalting step is necessary to adjust the buffer conditions prior to subsequent purification. Due to inherent limitations of SEC, the sample volume should be small in comparison to the column size. As a consequence, SEC is more often used as one of the last steps of a purification procedure for a recombinant protein.

Affinity chromatography is an efficient means of purifying recombinant proteins. Being expensive and potentially susceptible to degradation, it is often used in combination with IEC as the last step of a purification scheme. Immunoaffinity is appropriate for such a separation since high selectivity for the targeted protein as opposed to the bulk of the contaminating proteins is possible. However, as is the case for protein A or protein G, it is difficult to implement such bioaffinity procedures or to develop cleaning procedures which do not affect capacity. The leaching of immunogenic particles must be checked by sensitive, validated assays which must attest that the residual level is < 10 ppm, the current theoretical limit approved by Regulatory organizations.

FVIII has been isolated from fermenter harvests through a multi-step purification process which combines chromatography and diafiltration/ultrafiltration. The chromatographic steps used for one of the products (from Miles Laboratories) presently under clinical trials involve IEC, immunoaffinity using anti-FVIII mAb and SEC. This chromatographic series was designed to eliminate cell substrates, DNA, cellular proteins, endogenous or adventitious viruses, along with murine IgG originating from the immunoaffinity step.

CONCLUSION: FUTURE PROSPECTS

Chromatography has already been shown to be an effective and versatile improvement over conventional techniques in plasma fractionation. Its use has allowed the production of plasma derivatives with improved purity and safety, and has made possible the isolation of a new generation of derivatives. Chromatography will likely play an ever-increasing role in plasma fractionation. IEC and, to a lesser extent, SEC will probably remain basic separation methods in the near future.

Bioengineers will certainly encourage a broader use of affinity chromatography because it is more efficient than other techniques, provided that the chemical stability, reproducibility and non-toxicity of affinity sorbents is demonstrated. While mAb purification may appear necessary for the purification of recombinant proteins, its long-term interest in plasma fractionation remains questionable: it could be replaced by pseudo-affinity chromatography using non-biospecific ligands. There are already a number of plasma proteins that have been purified to homogeneity at the laboratory scale by taking advantage of the ability of, for example, dyes or lectins to act as analogues of specific ligands. Synthetic analogues of biomolecules could circumvent the problems associated with mAb chromatography and reduce the cost while providing easier-to-handle affinity for the target protein. Immobilized metal-ion affinity chromatography could have similar applications in the purification of plasma-derived and recombinant proteins.

Efficiency of purification procedures to remove non-human contaminants from genetically engineered protein is mandatory. However, much progress could result from the recent possibility offered by gene fusion to design and synthesize proteins with new biochemical and biophysical properties (e.g. N-terminus polyarginine tails). The additional polypeptide tag on the target protein may facilitate its extraction from the host cells and make it possible to direct subsequent affinity, ion-exchange, hydrophobic, covalent and/or metal chelate separations.

In conclusion, it is more than likely that chromatography will remain a method of choice for the purification of plasma proteins. The unique selectivity afforded by this separation method combined with the ever-improving parameters of modern supports will assure chromatography a secure position in the future of large-scale downstream processing of proteins.

FURTHER READING

Burnouf, T. (1991) Integration of chromatography with traditional plasma protein fractionation methods. *Bioseparation*, **1**, 383–396.

Curling, J.M. (1980) *Methods of Plasma Protein Fractionation*. Academic Press, London. 326 pp.

Kahn, R.A., Allen, R.W. and Baldassare, J. (1985) Alternative sources and substitutes for therapeutic blood components. *Blood*, **66**, 1–12.

Sene, C. and Boschetti, E. (1988) Downstream processes: equipment and techniques. In: *Advances in Biotechnological Processes*, **8** (Ed. A. Mizrahi), pp. 206–240.

Smit-Sibinga, C.Th., Das, P.C. and Seidl, S. (1985) *Plasma Fractionation and Blood Transfusion*. Martinus Nijhoff Publishers, Boston. 242 pp.

6 Novel Coagulation Factor Products

C.V. PROWSE

Haemostasis and coagulation

The formation of a clot, composed of the protein fibrin, involves reactions between about 20 plasma glycoproteins. *In vivo*, this process occurs at the same time as the aggregation of cells known as 'platelets', to form a plug or thrombus composed of varying amounts of fibrin, platelets, and trapped red cells. Normally this is then slowly degraded away by the enzymes of the fibrinolytic system (see Chapter 7). While it is increasingly apparent that haemostasis takes place on the surface of cells – such as platelets and the endothelial cells lining blood vessels – and requires their active participation, these are not considered in any detail in this chapter. It is only in the area of individual proteins that molecular medicine has, so far, had any great impact on our ability to correct disorders of haemostasis.

The proposal that blood coagulation involves enzymes, acting on other proteins in blood, dates back to the beginning of the century. It was only in the 1960s that the basis of our current understanding of coagulation became clear. A more recent interpretation of this is shown in Figure 6.1.

Most proteins involved in coagulation are assigned a roman numeral, and fall into three categories – proenzymes, cofactors and structural proteins. Coagulation involves the sequential conversion of proenzyme (e.g. Factor X) to enzyme (e.g. Factor Xa, the suffix 'a' denoting an active enzyme), which then converts the next proenzyme (Factor II or prothrombin), usually with the help of a cofactor (e.g. Factor V). These processes require the presence of calcium and an appropriate phospholipid suface, usually provided *in vivo* by the surface of activated cells.

Conventionally, coagulation has been divided into intrinsic and extrinsic paths, the latter so named as it involves a lipoprotein cofactor, tissue factor, not normally present in blood. Although this distinction has been helpful in interpreting laboratory assays it is apparent that this division may be misleading. Deficiency of the 'intrinsic' cofactor, Factor VIII, leads to bleeding. Normal haemostasis obviously requires both pathways, a finding currently

Plasma and Recombinant Blood Products in Medical Therapy
Edited by C.V. Prowse.   Published 1992 by John Wiley & Sons Ltd

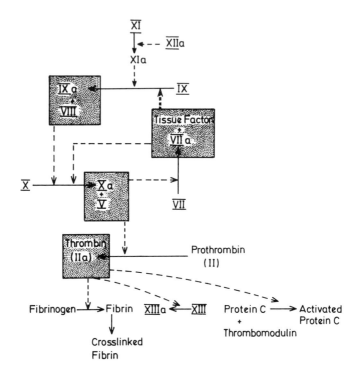

Fig. 6.1. *Coagulation mechanisms.* Most reactions also require the presence of calcium and a phospholipid surface to occur at an appropriate rate. Pro-enzymes are converted to enzymes, denoted by the suffix 'a'. Control occurs by inhibition of the enzyme components (e.g. IXa and Xa) by antithrombin, or degradation of cofactors (e.g. V or VIII) by activated protein C in combination with protein S. Thrombin, and possibly Factor Xa, also enhances the rate of coagulation by activation of the co-factors. Fibrin is eventually degraded by the fibrinolytic system (Chapter 7). Shaded boxes show the formation of multiprotein complexes, e.g. Xa and V, with calcium and phospholipid, from the prothrombinase complex

explained by the fact that Factor VIIa can activate Factor IX, as well as Factor X, whereas Factor XIa activation of Factor IX may be less important. Factor XI deficiency is not necessarily associated with bleeding.

Coagulation can be considered as a series of reactions each involving a complex of proteins bound, through calcium bridges, to the phopholipid surface of a cell. Figure 6.2 shows one example – the 'tenase' complex – in which Factor IXa (enzyme) and Factor VIII (cofactor) interact to activate Factor X (substrate). Although Factor IXa alone can slowly activate Factor X, the presence of calcium, phospholipid and Factor VIII accelerate the reaction several hundred thousand-fold and are absolutely required for adequate haemostasis. Deficiency of Factor VIII (haemophilia A) or Factor IX (haemophilia B) results in a life-long bleeding disorder.

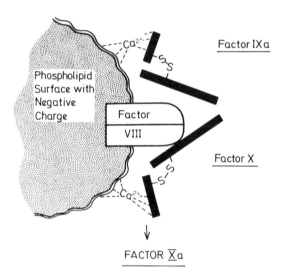

Fig. 6.2. The 'tenase' complex. Calcium-dependent binding of Factors IXa and X, and calcium-independent Factor VIII binding to a negatively charged phospholipid surface brings these various components together and lead to the activation of Factor X. Corresponding complexes occur at the other stages of coagulation

Obviously coagulation must be limited or the continued action of coagulant enzyme–cofactor complexes would rapidly clot all available blood. This is achieved at two levels – degradation of the cofactors and inhibition of the enzymes. The former involves thrombin activation of protein C with the participation of the endothelial cell cofactor thrombomodulin. Activated protein C and another plasma protein, protein S, then act on the cofactors V and VIII to degrade them. Proteins C and S are structurally very similar to the pro-enzymes involved in coagulation.

Inhibition of enzymes is accomplished by glycoproteins present in plasma. Most of these belong to a structurally similar family of proteins, the serpins (serine protease inhibitors). A distinct inhibitor, extrinsic path inhibitor (EPI) or lipoprotein-associated coagulation inhibitor (LACI), controls the action of the Factor VIIa tissue factor complex. The major inhibitor of most coagulant enzymes is the serpin, antithrombin-III. The action of this, and some other serpins, is greatly enhanced by heparin, a highly sulphated polysaccharide.

As would be expected, deficiency of the proteins involved in inhibition of coagulation, e.g. protein C or antithrombin-III, results in excess coagulation. Patients with such deficiencies present with recurrent thrombosis rather than the lifelong bleeding disorders associated with deficiency of the pro-coagulant proteins. In either case the obvious therapy is to replace the missing protein. Table 6.1 lists the more common deficiency states.

Table 6.1 Congenital deficiencies of haemostatic and related proteins

Symptoms	Protein involved	Deficiency	Frequency
Bleeding	Factor VIII	Haemophilia A	1:10000*
	Factor IX	Haemophilia B	1:60000*
	von Willebrand Factor	von Willebrand's disease	1:5000*
Thrombosis	Antithrombin III	Recurrent thrombosis	1:5000*
	Protein C	Recurrent thrombosis	1:15000**
	Protein S	Recurrent thrombosis	1:15000**
Lung disease	α_1– Protease inhibitor	Emphysema	1:3000*

* Rate of gene defect; not all require routine therapy.
** Represents estimates of patients presenting with symptoms for treatment. More have genetic defects not requiring routine therapy.

During the 1960s and 1970s many of the proteins mentioned above were isolated and their structure fully described. At the same time the preparation of coagulation factor concentrates from human plasma, enabling replacement therapy of the more common deficiency states, was developed (see Chapter 3). The importance of this should not be underestimated. For the first time haemophiliacs, for example, could lead an almost normal life with the expectation of a full lifespan.

Although concentrates of Factor VIII were developed during this period, a full description of its structure resisted the conventional approach of protein purification and analysis, partly due to its instability and low concentration in plasma. With the cloning of the Factor VIII gene in 1984, these matters were clarified. Now, the genes for most of the proteins involved in coagulation have been characterized. A summary of these is given in Appendix 2 at the end of the book.

Here we also consider α_1-protease inhibitor (α_1-PI or antitrypsin). While deficiency of this protein is usually associated with lung disease, it is structurally very similar to antithrombin and is involved in haemostasis as an inhibitor of activated protein C, Factor XIa and possibly Xa. Concentrates of α_1-PI are also available from human plasma and the similarity of antithrombin and antitrypsin genes suggests approaches to therapy using genetic manipulation, that apply to both deficiency states.

DISADVANTAGES OF CONVENTIONAL THERAPEUTIC PRODUCTS

Conventional products, for the treatment of the deficiency states listed above, are protein concentrates prepared from the obvious source, human plasma collected by Transfusion Services or commercial organizations. They contain a large number of other proteins in addition to the one of interest, especially in concentrates of proteins present at low concentrations in normal plasma, such as Factor VIII.

However, all these are native, human proteins. In addition they may contain microorganisms, such as viruses, derived from infected blood donors. This can be a greater problem with paid, rather than volunteer donors, and all blood-collection agencies now make considerable efforts to exclude any infected donations.

While it was recognized that blood products could transmit disease many years ago, the advent of the AIDS epidemic and the transmission of AIDS by blood products, such as Factor VIII in the early 1980s, demanded immediate action. It was known that pasteurization (heating in solution at 60°C for 10 h) inactivated viruses, but at that time this approach resulted in large losses of the more labile proteins, such as Factor VIII. As the raw material (human plasma) is limited, the effect of loss of yield could be a limited

Table 6.2 Pathogenic viruses of interest: plasma – derived products

Virus	Type	Envelope	Disease	Susceptibility		
				SHT	P	SD
Human immunodeficiency virus (HIV)	RNA/SS	+	AIDS	+	+	+
Hepatitis B virus (HBV)	DNA/DS	+	Hepatitis	+	+	+
Hepatitis D virus (HDV)	RNA/SS	+	± Hepatoma	NT†	NT	NT
Hepatitis C virus* (HCV)	RNA/SS	+		+	+	+
B19 Parvovirus	DNA/SS	–	Fifth disease	±	?	–

Viruses are classified by whether they have a genome of RNA or DNA which is single- (SS) or double- (DS) stranded, and whether or not they have a lipid envelope. Susceptibility to viral inactivation procedures is shown for severe heat treatment (80°C for 72h) of freeze-dried material (SHT), pasteurization (P) (60°C for 10h) in solution or solvent detergent (SD) treatment (1% Tween-80, 0.3% tri-N-butyl phosphate at 25°C for 6h) in solution.

* Non-A, non-B hepatitis is a disease of concern. While most transfusion-transmitted cases appear to be due to HCV, some may be due to an uncharacterized virus. HDV is a defective virus requiring prior HBV infection to allow its expression. Effective vaccines are available for HBV.

† NT: not tested.

supply of a life-saving product. For this, and other reasons, most manufacturers initially used heat treatment of the freeze-dried final product, to inactivate viruses. If this is done for long enough at high enough temperatures, it is certainly sufficient to inactivate human immunodeficiency virus (HIV) and other viruses of concern (Table 6.2). This approach has the advantage that it is done on the final product and thus eliminates the possibility of re-contamination of the product during further processing. However, further purification may be necessary to remove proteins that might otherwise render the product poorly soluble after heating.

Most manufacturers now use either pasteurization or treatment with a mixture of solvent and detergent to inactivate viruses, together with viral elimination by the protein purification process. Pasteurization usually requires further purification of the product to remove contaminating proteins together with use of additives, such as sugars, to protect the protein of interest during heating. Solvent detergent (SD) is milder but requires subsequent removal of the toxic reagents. SD is only effective for enveloped viruses. Fortunately the important known pathogenic viruses all fall into this group (Table 6.2).

The second result of the AIDS epidemic was that the subsequent detailed evaluation of haemophiliac patients revealed that their immune system was suppressed. For example, they did not mount a normal antibody response. This effect was seen whether or not the patients were infected with the AIDS virus and was apparent in both Factor VIII and IX deficiency. On the basis of some laboratory results it has been suggested that this may be due to the regular infusion of contaminating proteins in the therapeutic concentrates. Despite extensive attempts to demonstrate this clinically, by comparing patients receiving different purity concentrates, there is no clinical evidence to support this hypothesis. Such studies are long and difficult to perform. Even in the absence of such clinical evidence, there is an increasing demand for higher purity concentrates. The move towards products with less contaminant protein had already begun due to the requirements of heat treatment or pasteurization. For Factor IX products there is a good scientific basis for the move towards a purer product. Conventional Factor IX products have been associated with inappropriate thrombosis in a small number of patients, particularly those with liver disease. Use of higher purity products reduces this risk.

The production of therapeutic products by biotechnology would appear to offer a solution to many of the disadvantages of plasma derived products. Potentially such an approach could provide an unlimited supply of pure product with no risk of infection from an occasional infected donor. The latter risk has now been minimized by the introduction of viral inactivation procedures for plasma-derived products. The risk of contamination also exists for recombinant products as they are produced from cell cultures that are susceptible to infection. This can also be minimized by screening of the stock culture, which is easier to control than for thousands of donors, and product. A second concern is the need to extensively purify the recombinant product. These are usually produced in non-human cells and it is essential to remove all traces of protein arising from the host cell or culture medium. The third main concern for recombinant products is whether an entirely native product is made. If not, it may be seen as foreign by the patient and induce an immune response. Such structural changes might arise by inappropriate folding of the protein backbone or by inappropriate addition of other structures to the protein backbone. For example, all coagulation factors are glycoproteins in which carbohydrate side-chains are added to the protein after synthesis. The type of carbohydrate added depends on the type of cell in which the protein is made. Bacterial cells may add no carbohydrate and yeast a different type of carbohydrate than mammalian cells. Some concern in this area has resulted from the recent observation that recombinant Factor VIII may induce a higher than normal frequency of antibodies in previously untreated haemophiliacs. This evidence is only preliminary as it is based on a small group of patients. Even if it does not induce antibodies, subtle changes in structure of recombinant proteins (e.g. a reduced content of the carbohydrate group sialic acid) are known to affect the half-life of the protein after transfusion.

FACTOR VIII AND VON WILLEBRAND FACTOR

PROTEIN AND GENE STRUCTURE

Factor VIII is only present at very low concentrations in plasma, about 200 ng/ml or 0.003% of total plasma protein. Deficiency occurs in about 1 in 10 000 of the population, of which about one-third are new mutations. In its most severe form the resultant haemophilia A is a life-long bleeding disorder which leads to severe disability, including joint deterioration, and early death, but which is completely reversible by replacement therapy with Factor VIII. Except for very rare cases, the deficiency only occurs in males as the gene is on the X chromosome.

In blood, Factor VIII circulates as a complex with the multimeric protein von Willebrand factor (vWf) which prolongs the half-life of Factor VIII. Deficiency of von Willebrand factor thus also results in deficiency of Factor VIII as, although the patient can make Factor VIII, it is rapidly lost from the circulation. Although vWf may participate in the synthesis and stabilization of Factor VIII (see below) it does not actively participate in coagulation. It is involved in haemostasis as it is required for the adhesion of platelets at sites of injury. It may thus localize Factor VIII, and hence coagulation, to such sites. Unlike Factor VIII, vWf deficiency is seen in both men and women, as the gene is found on chromosome 12.

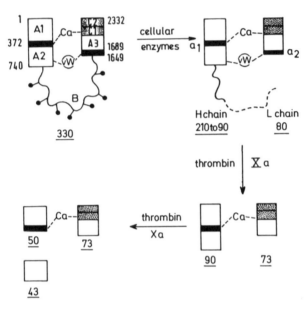

Fig. 6.3. The structure of Factor VIII. Factor VIII is initially synthesized as a single chain molecule of 330000 Da with an A1.A1.B.A3.C1.C2 domain structure. Amino acid residue locations are shown in small numbers. The highly glycosylated (●) B domain is partially degraded prior to secretion yielding heavy and light chains of 210 to 90 and 80 kDa, respectively, held together by calcium (Ca) and von Willebrand factor (vW). Thrombin (or Xa) cleaves this adjacent to highly acidic regions (a_1 and a_2 shown in black) to yield fully active Factor VIII, with loss of vWf binding. Activated protein C inactivates the molecule by cleavage at residue 336, and Factor Xa at residue 1721

Due to difficulties in purifying Factor VIII its structure did not become fully apparent until after the cloning of the Factor VIII gene in 1984. The gene occupies about 0.1% of the X chromosome or 186000 bases, and contains 26 exons coding for a mature protein of 2332 amino acids. This is composed of three A domains followed by two C domains with a large intervening B domain between the A2 and A3 structure (Figure 6.3).

The molecule contains sulphate groups and is heavily glycosylated, mainly in the B domain. The B domain shows considerable variation between species and is also different from the equivalent portion of Factor V, which is otherwise fairly similar in structure. In fact, the B domain is not required for Factor VIII activity, although it does appear to be involved in its synthesis (see below). Apart from the homology with equivalent structures in factor V, the A and C domains show similarities with parts of ceruloplasmin, a human copper-binding protein, and discoidin, a lipid-binding protein from slime moulds. These may be involved in the binding of Factor VIII to metal ions and phospholipid, respectively. The binding sites for Factor IXa and Factor X are not yet known, but the binding to vWf requires a highly acidic region on the N-terminal side of the A3 domain. A similar acidic region is found between the A1 and A2 domains. Both contain sulphated tyrosine groups and are adjacent to the sites of the activation of Factor VIII by thrombin.

While the Factor VIII gene encodes a single chain protein, it becomes degraded within the B domain prior to secretion and in plasma is found as a dimer of an 80 kD light chain and a variable length heavy chain (90–210 kD) held together by calcium ions (Figure 6.3).

These forms have minimal activity in coagulation and need to be cleaved by thrombin (or Factor Xa) to express their full activity. Thrombin cleaves the molecule after arginine residues at positions 372, 740 and 1689. The cleavage at residue 740, leading to loss of any residual B domain, is not essential. Recombinant technology has shown that mutations at arginine-372 or -1689 results in inactive Factor VIII and cleavage at both residues is thus required for full activity. The latter results in loss of the second acid domain, loss of affinity for vWf and reduction in size of the light chain. There is some controversy as to whether the fully active form of Factor VIII is a dimer of 73 kD-degraded light chain with 90 kD heavy chain, or a heterotrimer in which the heavy chain has been degraded to 50 kD and 43 kD fragments. The consensus is in favour of the latter. In any case, the heterotrimer is not stable due to dissociation of the 43 kD heavy chain portion from the complex, possibly in association with vWf. Factor VIII is also inactivated by enzymic degradation, for example by the action of activated protein C after arginine-336 in the heavy chain. Mutation of this residue to alanine, making it resistant to protein C, results in a more stable activated Factor VIII. Analysis of Factor VIII concentrates shows different patterns of the sizes of heavy-chain component in various products.

The gene for vWf contains 52 exons. It encodes a protein of which only the C-terminal 2050 amino acids form vWf. The N-terminal portion of this precursor protein is involved in the polymerization of vWf but is cleaved from it, to form vWf antigen-II, prior to secretion. Unlike Factor VIII, which is largely made in the liver, vWf is mainly synthesized by endothelial cells with some contribution from platelets. The 220 kD subunit of vWf has a domain structure in which binding sites, for Factor VIII, platelet glycoproteins Ib/IX and IIb/IIIa, collagen, heparin and fibrin have been identified (Figure 6.4). These are required for the activity of vWf in promoting platelet–subendothelial and platelet–platelet binding during haemostasis. Even though each subunit contains the appropriate binding site for these activities, effective function is only seen in large polymers of the vWf subunit with molecular weights in the $2\text{–}10 \times 10^6$ Da range. Such polymerization occurs in an anti-parallel manner prior to secretion of the protein and does not occur if the portion of gene encoding vWf antigen-II is deleted.

Analysis of current Factor VIII concentrates shows most contain some vWf, although this is minimal in the more highly purified concentrates.

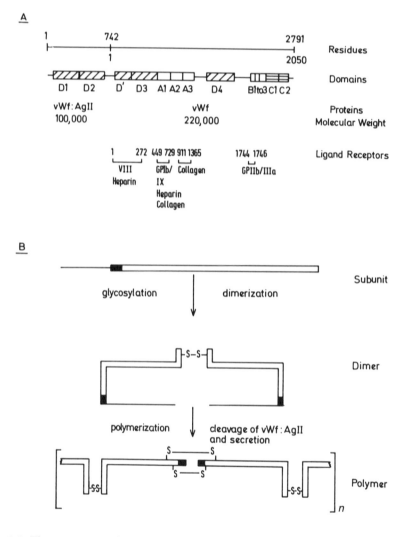

Fig. 6.4. The structures of von Willebrand Factor subunits and polymers. (A) Structure of vWf and vWf:AgII. A, B, C and D are domains repeated within the molecule. Regions involved in binding to various ligands are also shown. GPIb/IX and GPIIb/IIIa refer to areas involved in binding to specific glycoproteins (GP) on platelets. (B) Mode of formation of vWf dimers and subsequent polymerization during synthesis and secretion

Clinical studies suggest that those concentrates containing the higher polymers are most effective in reducing bleeding time in patients with von Willebrand's disease. Those that only contain lower vWf polymers or contain minimal vWf are of little use for such therapy.

Table 6.3 Newer plasma-derived Factor VIII/vWf products

Product	Company	Chromatography process	Specific activity** (U/mg)	Albumin added	vWf activity
Hemofil M*	Baxter	F$_{VIII}$ antibody	> 2000 (10)	+	Low
Monoclate P	Armour	vWf antibody	> 2000 (10)	+	Low
Octa-VI*	Octapharma	Anion exchange	100–200	–	+
VHP-VIII*	Biotransfusion	Anion exchange	100–200	–	+
VIII: CP	Behring/Novo ?	Anion exchange	100–200 (?)	+	?
Koate: HP*	Cutter	Gel filtration	50 (10)	+	?
FVIII: HP*	Baden Red Cross	Gel filtration	50 (8)	+	?
(Unnamed)*	Alpha	'Affinity'	? 50	?	?
VHP-vWf*	Biotransfusion	Anion exchange	100 (for vWf)	–	+

* The viral inactivation step used is solvent detergent (*) or pasteurization.

** Specific activities in parentheses represents values after albumin addition.

+/– denotes presence/absence of albumin or vWf activity in individual products.

NOVEL PLASMA-DERIVED FACTOR VIII/vWf PRODUCT

With the development of effective methods to inactivate viruses in plasma-derived products, the main thrust in developing novel plasma derived Factor VIII/vWf concentrates has moved towards products of higher purity. Conventional precipitation-based technology (Chapter 3) has been unable to yield products with a specific activity much greater than 10 U/mg. This must be viewed against a knowledge that pure Factor VIII has a specific activity > 2000 U/mg and pure vWf > 100 U/mg.

The new generation of products all make use of some form of chromatography. These fall into two categories – conventional chromatography and purification based on the use of monoclonal antibodies (Table 6.3). Two forms of the latter have been developed. One makes use of a Factor VIII monoclonal antibody to Factor VIII directly, the other uses a vWf antibody to capture vWf/VIII complex, with subsequent recovery of the Factor VIII by elution with calcium, leaving the majority of the vWf on the column (see Chapter 5). Either methods yields essentially pure Factor VIII of 2000 to 3000 U/mg, although it has been found necessary to add back albumin to stabilize the product. The final specific activity is thus only 5–10 U/mg.

Alternatively, application of conventional chromatographic methods, such as size-exclusion chromatography, anion-exchange chromatography (in combination with a large pore gels to improve capacity) or 'affinity' chromatography, has yielded concentrates with specific activities in the 10–200 U/mg range, i.e. up to 10% pure. The advantages of such products are that they are cheaper to prepare and may retain high-molecular-weight vWf polymers. A separate vWf concentrate can also be prepared by this approach (see Chapter 5).

RECOMBINANT PRODUCTS

Two Factor VIII recombinant products have been at clinical trial for at least the last two years. So far, these have proven to be safe and effective, apart from the concern over induction of inhibitors in previously untreated patients already mentioned. Both these have been made by insertion of cDNA encoding the entire Factor VIII protein into mammalian cells. The chief problem has been the low level of expression and the instability of the Factor VIII once secreted. Some of the reasons for this have been elucidated. Firstly, the level of messenger RNA (mRNA) for Factor VIII is low. This may be partly due to large size of the gene. Secondly, once produced the Factor VIII follows the usual secretory pathway of entry into the endoplasmic reticulum. Here much of it associates with a resident protein known as BiP (immunoglobulin heavy-chain binding protein) or GRP78. Thirdly, the instability of Factor VIII following secretion has been shown to result from degradation of the heavy chain. This can be avoided by adding vWf which promotes association between heavy and light chains. This may be accomplished by addition of serum or

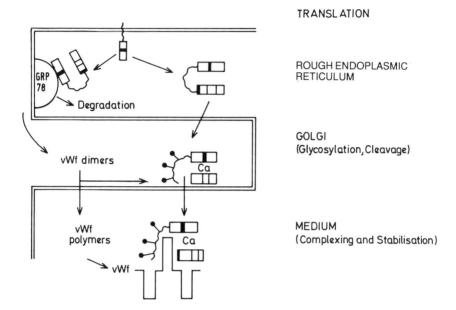

Fig. 6.5. Synthesis of Factor VIII–von Willebrand Factor. Much of the nascent Factor rVIII polypeptide binds GRP78 in the rough endoplasmic reticulum and is recycled. The remaining Factor VIII is subjected to post-translational modification in the Golgi apparatus. During secretion from here, vWf promotes correct association of Factor VIII heavy and light chains. vWf polymerization occurs in the same compartments. The complex of vWf and Factor VIII protects the heavy chain of Factor VIII from degradation after secretion. The symbol ——● denotes carbohydrate side chains

vWf or preferably by co-expression of vWf and Factor VIII in the chosen cell line to mimic the natural process (Figure 6.5).

Other improvements have involved attempts to reduce the level of GRP78 using anti-sense nucleic acid, improving the levels of RNA by use of inducible vectors and careful selection of cell lines. Different mammalian cell lines transfected with the same Factor VIII construct are known to vary by as much as five- to ten-fold in their secretion of Factor VIII. Current work has centred on the use of chinese hamster ovary (CHO) and baby hamster kidney (BHK) cells. Expression levels are of the order of 1–10 IU (0.2–2 µg) per million cells and purification is based on the use of monoclonal antibodies.

An alternative approach has been to make use of cDNA that does not encode the B domain. Both co-expression of separate heavy and light chains, and use of a single B domain-deleted structure have been assessed with the latter appearing more hopeful. Deletion of the entire B domain from residue 740 onwards is allowable and this can even be extended up to residue 1666 in the terminal acid region of the light chain. Further extension of the deletion results in a reduced binding of vWf and is not desirable. Factor VIII produced from such constructs is fully active and is expressed at levels five-to ten-fold higher than for the full size protein. Such increases may relate partly to the reduced mRNA size but are also based on the finding that intracellular degradation of the nascent protein via the GRP78 path is reduced. Substitution of the B domain of Factor V into the Factor VIII gene, in place of the normal B domain, has also been assessed by recombinant methods. This results in a product with Factor VIII activity that is produced at two- or three-fold the level of normal Factor VIII.

While the cDNA for vWf has been characterized and use made of it in studying the expression of recombinant Factor VIII, this has only recently been accomplished. Preparation of a recombinant therapeutic vWf would require considerably more work. Patient trials, if they are considered appropriate, are some years away.

FUTURE DIRECTIONS: TRANSGENIC ANIMALS, GENE THERAPY AND TRANSPLANTATION

With the levels of product obtained with current technology, preparation of any recombinant product, such as Factor VIII, requires a large fermentation facility. An alternative possibility is provided by transgenic animals. In this technique the gene of interest is injected directly into the fertile egg which is then placed in a surrogate mother and eventually can yield an animal in which all the cells contain the inserted gene. By placing the gene in a suitable framework of DNA, prior to injection, it becomes possible to obtain high-level tissue-specific expression of the gene. Thus, in theory, it is possible to direct sheep or cows to produce high levels of foreign protein in their milk. While this has yet to be done for Factor VIII, considerable progress has been made for Factor IX and α_1-protease inhibitor. This approach has the advantage of being renewable and relatively cheap to maintain (after the initial development) compared to cell culture. Transgenic animals can produce offspring with the same characteristics. However, like cell culture, this approach only provides a treatment not a cure. A cure would require insertion of the appropriate gene into the deficient patient – gene therapy. Currently, the most hopeful approach makes use of modified retrovirus to insert the appropriate gene into the target cells. Lymphocytes, marrow, fibroblasts and endothelial cells have been studied, but to date protein synthesis has been at low levels and of limited duration. Despite this, the first human trial has commenced with the aim of curing the fatal deficiency of adenosine deaminase. With the available therapies it is likely to be at least ten years before such an approach will be considered for haemophilia. A more likely alternative in the immediate future is liver transplantation. This has been undertaken to treat acute liver failure in haemophiliacs and is known to cure Factor VIII deficiency. With the improving success of this operation and the recent successful partial liver transplantation from a live mother to her baby, this approach is increasingly feasible. One should note, however, that while this cures the patient it does not eliminate the defective gene which will be passed on to his offspring. The same applies to 'somatic' gene therapy.

TREATMENT OF INHIBITOR PATIENTS

Between 5 and 20% of severe haemophiliacs eventually develop antibodies to the Factor VIII used to treat them. These can often be overcome by giving very high doses of Factor VIII but this may induce a further rise in antibody level, unless continued for a period of months. The patient may then become tolerant and cease producing antibody.

Apart from the potential improved availability of native Factor VIIII, biotechnology offers a number of possible therapies for such patients. For instance, most inhibitory antibodies are directed to the C domain or acid-rich regions of Factor VIII. Recombinant fragments of Factor VIII or synthetic peptides corresponding to these regions could be used to block the antibodies, allowing conventional Factor VIII therapy, or to induce tolerance. Such patients are already treated with activated prothrombin complex concentrates, which are effective in preventing bleeding in around two-thirds of cases. This is thought to occur through induction of coagulation by a Factor VIII-independent path. This has given rise to three possible novel approaches. The first, and most advanced, involves the use of recombinant Factor VIIa or the equivalent plasma-derived product. Ongoing clinical trials suggest this also is effective in about two-thirds of patients. While very high doses are required, no adverse effects (such as inappropriate coagulation) have been reported in patients and the product does not induce any further increase in Factor VIII inhibitor. High levels of Factor VIIa have been shown to directly activate Factor X, albeit inefficiently. The mechanism of action in patients is more likely to involve formation of a Factor X-activating complex with exposed tissue factor at the site of injury.

The other two alternatives involve the use of recombinant tissue factor apoprotein or conventionally purified Factor Xa and phospholipid. These have been shown to be effective in animals with haemophilia, but have yet to be assessed in patients. There is some doubt that these will be undertaken as the difference between the doses required to stop bleeding and those resulting in systemic activation of coagulation are less than one would desire.

FACTOR IX

PROTEIN AND GENE STRUCTURE

Deficiency of Factor IX, haemophilia B, results in symptoms identical to those of haemophilia A. The gene is also found on the X chromosome, although the frequency of the defect is rather lower. The structure of the protein was established by conventional protein chemistry prior to the cloning of the gene in 1982. Factor IX is a single-chain glycoprotein of molecular

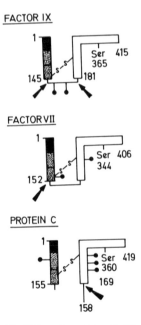

Fig. 6.6. Structure of Factors IX, VII and protein C. The homologous domain structure of these three vitamin K-dependent pro-enzymes is indicated. The numbers refer to the sequence of amino acids, with the active site serine (Ser) residue of the protease domain indicated. Glycosylation sites and interchain disulphide bonds are represented. Activation occurs at the positions indicated by arrows on the single or two (protein C) chain pro-enzyme with release of an activation peptide (not Factor VII) to yield the two-chain disulphide-linked active enzyme. Key: ■, GLA domain; ▨, EGF domain; ———, activation peptide; □, protease domain; →, cleavage to yield enzyme; ———●, carbohydrate side chains; –S–S–, interchain disulphide bond

weight 57 000 (415 amino acids) synthesized in the liver. During coagulation, it is activated by cleavage at two points (residues 145 and 180) releasing a carbohydrate-rich activation peptide and yielding the two-chain active enzyme, Factor IXa (Figure 6.6). Activation occurs by the same pathway whether it is caused by Factor XIa or Factor VIIa–tissue factor complex. The heavy chain of Factor IXa has a structure equivalent to that of trypsin, with a serine active site. This part of the molecule thus provides the enzymic activity of Factor IXa in cleaving Factor X. The light chain of Factor IXa is also required for activity. It is composed of three domains. Two of these are homologous to epidermal growth factor and are required for activity but are of uncertain function. They are involved in calcium binding and may provide receptors for endothelial cells and Factor VIII. The N-terminal domain is known as the GLA domain, as it contains 12 γ-carboxylglutamic acid (GLA) residues. These residues are involved in the calcium-dependent binding of Factors IX and IXa to phospholipid surfaces, which is essential for full activity. The conversion of these glutamic acid residues to GLA residues occurs after synthesis, but prior to secretion of the protein from the liver. It requires the action of a vitamin K-dependent carboxylase and if this enzyme cannot act, due to vitamin K deficiency or inhibition by coumarin drugs such as warfarin, a non-carboxylated and essentially inactive Factor IX is produced. Corresponding reactions take place for the other vitamin K-dependent pro-enzymes involved in blood coagulation: Factors II (prothrombin), VII and X, protein C and protein S, all of which have similar structures (Figure 6.6). Carboxylation only occurs on glutamic acids in the N-terminal region of these proteins, not on glutamate residues elsewhere in the molecule. These reactions are dependent on binding of the vitamin K-dependent carboxylase to a propeptide region, cleaved from the N-terminal of the protein prior to secretion.

The light chain of Factor IX also contains a β-hydroxyl group on aspartic acid-60 in the first epidermal growth factor (EGF) domain. As with the carboxylation reaction, addition of the hydroxy group and of carbohydrate chains to the activation peptide region of Factor IX occurs after synthesis of the protein backbone and is not under the control of the Factor IX gene. Such post-translational modifications have resulted in problems in preparing recombinant Factor IX.

It is apparent from Figure 6.6 that the structures of the vitamin K-dependent coagulation factors are similar but differences also exist, as is obvious from their unique specificities. Apart from these differences in binding and cleavage of substrates, other properties of this family of proteins also diverge. Amongst these are their ability to bind heparin (or dextran sulphate) and copper chromatography gels. Unlike other members of the family, Factor IX (and in the case of copper gels, protein C) shows high affinity for both types of gel. This property has been utilized in preparation of purer Factor IX products. Factor VII may be separated from other proteins of this group by conventional anion-exchange chromatography, for which it has a lower affinity.

The Factor IX gene is found on the X chromosome but is located closer to the centromere than that for Factor VIII. It spans 34 000 nucleotides including 8 exons encoding a mRNA of 2800 bases.

PLASMA-DERIVED CONCENTRATES

Conventional plasma concentrates of Factor IX are prepared by DEAE anion-exchange chromatography of plasma. Due to their similar properties, Factors II and X, protein C and protein S (and in some cases Factor VII) are also concentrated in these preparations which are also known as three (II, IX, X) or four (II, VII, IX, X) factor prothrombin complex concentrates (PCC).

Such products can be further purified by affinity chromatography on heparin, dextran sulphate or copper gels or by immunoaffinity chromatography using monoclonal antibody to Factor IX. The specific activity of these products can be as high as 200 U/mg (Table 6.4) indicating that they contain little protein other than Factor IX. *In vivo* studies, in animals and patients, with these high-purity products show them to be effective in controlling bleeding and to have a reduced risk or inducing thrombosis or intravascular coagulation. The latter side-effect is associated with conventional PCCs, particularly when they are used at high doses or in patients with liver disease. As many haemophiliacs have chronic liver disease due to infection with hepatitis virus prior to the introduction virus-inactivation steps in blood product manufacture, the high-purity products are likely to be increasingly in demand for the treatment of haemophilia B.

All the vitamin K-dependent proteins are made in the liver and liver disease may result in bleeding problems due to reduced synthesis. Despite the risks, PCC have been used to treat bleeding in such patients and also following coumarin-induced inhibition of synthesis of the same protein family. High-purity Factor IX products will be of no use in such patients as the requirement is to replace all the absent coagulation factors.

RECOMBINANT PRODUCTS

Although the Factor IX gene was cloned in 1982, progress in developing a recombinant product has been slow. This is partly because of the lower demand for the product – there are only about 1000 patients in the United Kingdom – and partly due to the multiple post-translational modifications in Factor IX. These include carboxylation, hydroxylation, glycosylation and sulphation of the nascent protein.

Initial studies showed that while low levels of fully active recombinant product could be produced from cDNA constructs, attempts to increase expression levels often resulted in respectable levels of protein synthesis but with very low activity. This was shown to be due to inadequate carboxylation of the N-terminal glutamic acid residues. Subsequently careful choice of cell lines, presumably to yield cells with appropriate carboxylase activity, together with vitamin K and bicarbonate supplementation of culture media yielded fully carboxylated products at high levels.

One outcome of this work was the finding that interaction of the nascent protein with the carboxylase occurred via the pro-peptide of vitamin K-dependent proteins. This pro-peptide is cleaved from the protein during secretion. By engineering changes at individual positions in this region, the area between residues -18 and -5 have been shown to be involved in this interaction (Table 6.5). This is confirmed by the description of haemophilia B patients with mutations in this region.

A further requirement for full activity of recombinant Factor IX is cleavage of the pro-peptide. This involves residues at -5, -1 and 1 (Table 6.5). Factor IX is unusual in having a tyrosine rather than alanine at position $+1$, the N-terminal of the plasma protein. Recent studies indicate that mutation of this

Table 6.4 High-purity Factor IX concentrate

Product	Company	Chromatography process	Specific activity (U/mg)	Comment
VHP-IX	Biotransfusion	Anion exchange + heparin	> 100	
Factor IX	Baxter/Red Cross	Anion exchange + sulphated dextran	33	Contains Factor X
Mononine	Armour	Monoclonal antibody	> 100	
Alphanine	Alpha	Anion exchange, barium adsorption and dextran sulphate	70	Contains Factor X
(Unnamed)	Bioproducts Lab	Anion exchange + copper chelate	> 100	Contains protein C

Table 6.5 Structure of the propeptide region of vitamin K-dependent proteins

	-10					-5				-1	+1				+5				
IX	Ala	Asn	Lys	Ile	Leu	Asn	Arg	Pro	Lys	Arg	Tyr	Asn	Ser	Gly	Lys	Leu	GLA††	GLA	Phe
VII	*	His	Gly	Val	*	His	*	Arg	Arg	*	Ala	*	Ala	–	Phe	*	*	*	Leu
X	*	*	Asn	*	*	Ala	*	Val	Thr	*	Ala	*	*	–	Phe	*	*	*	Met
II	*	Arg	Ser	Leu	*	Gln	Ile	Val	Arg	*	Ala	*	Thr	–	Phe	*	*	*	Val
C	*	His	Gln	Val	*	Arg	Arg	Arg	*	*	Ale	*	*	–	Phe	*	*	*	Leu
S	*	Ser	Gln	Val	*	Val	*	Lys	Arg	*	Ala	*	*	–	Lys	*	*	*	Thr
IX var†	*	*	*	*	*	*	*	*	*	*	Ala	*	*	*	*	*	*	*	*
	g							c		c	c						g	g	

c: Involved in cleavage of propeptide.
g: involved in carboxylation reaction (also residues -18, -17, -16 and -15).
*: Identical residue to Factor IX.
†IX var: Recombinant Factor IX: Tyr-1 to Ala.
††GLA: γ-Carboxyglutamic acid.

residue to alanine allows production of an appropriately cleaved, fully carboxylated recombinant Factor IX of specific activity 200 U/mg from BHK cells at levels similar to those found in normal plasma. Parallel work has shown a similar level of product and specific activity using wild-type Factor IX cDNA and murine C127 cells. This study also examined the effect of exchanging the epidermal growth factor (EGF) domains of Factor IX for those of Factor X. Exchange of EGF1 had little effect, whereas swapping both EFG domains reduced specific activity but not 'Factor IX' synthesis. This implies EGF2 of Factor IX has a unique function in Factor IX, such as being involved in its interaction with Factor VIII. These changes had no effect on the extent of carboxylation or hydroxylation of the Factor IX compared to wild-type recombinant Factor IX. About half the molecules of recombinant Factor IXs were hydroxylated on the aspartate residue in EGF1, compared to 25% and 100% in plasma-derived Factors IX and X. Recombinant Factor IX has yet to be produced at a scale that would allow clinical trials. As in the case of Factor VIII alternative approaches to therapy or treatment are being sought.

The Factor IX gene has been transferred into various cells, such as fibroblasts, using retroviral vectors and it has been demonstrated that implanting such cells in rodents allows low level expression of Factor IX in plasma, at least for a period of weeks. Studies have now commenced on such 'gene therapy' in dogs with haemophilia B.

Transgenic sheep have been established which express human Factor IX in their milk using a β-lactoglobulin gene construct. These initial studies used a cDNA for Factor IX and resulted in very low levels of expression. Improved constructs using control and intron sequences from the genomic Factor IX DNA, and use of animals with multiple copies of the gene in transgenic mice suggest that higher level expression is achievable. Encouraging results have recently been obtained using cultured liver cells from such 'IX-transgenic' mice.

As for Factor VIII deficiency, liver transplantation can cure haemophilia B. This offers a more immediate hope of lifetime cure.

PROTEIN C AND OTHER VITAMIN K-DEPENDENT PROTEINS

Amongst these, progress on recombinant Factors IX and VII has already been described. All the other vitamin K-dependent proteins have been cloned (see Appendix 2) but only protein C is being actively assessed as a potential therapeutic product. Protein C has a similar structure to Factor IX (Figure 6.6) but following activation by thrombin and thrombomodulin, the activated protein is involved in degradation of Factors V and VIII. Deficiency of protein C is one of the more commonly identified causes of congenital recurrent thrombosis. Current treatment involves use of anticoagulants such as warfarin. There is no specific plasma-derived concentrate available, although PCCs contain elevated levels of protein C and have been used for replacement therapy. Laboratory studies have shown the feasibility of preparing protein C concentrate from PCC by affinity or immunoaffinity chromatography.

At least one commercial company has embarked on preparation of a recombinant protein C therapeutic. While similar problems exist for this product and Factor IX, progress has been more rapid and studies in animal models have commenced. These have indicated that protein C or activated protein C may be useful for patients other than those with congenital deficiency. Preliminary studies show that it may be useful in controlling disseminated intravascular coagulation, a syndrome involving chronic activation of the coagulation mechanism throughout the body. This occurs, for example, following bacterial infection of the blood (sepsis), a common event in traumatized patients. Replacement therapy with antithrombin-III (see below) may also be useful in this group. In addition, activated protein C also appears to be useful in promoting lysis of thrombi. How it achieves this is unclear. It may involve consumption of plasminogen activator inhibitors by activated protein C, effectively increasing the availability of active plasminogen activator (see Chapter 7).

Protein S might also be considered as a therapeutic product. Deficiency of this protein occurs at a frequency similar to protein C deficiency and results in a similar recurrent thrombosis. Protein S is unusual among the vitamin K-dependent proteins in that its C-terminal half is dissimilar to that of the other members of the family and has no known enzyme function. Protein S is inactivated by thrombin and about half of it normally circulates as a complex with C4b-binding protein, a regulatory component of the complement system. Only the unbound form of protein S is active in coagulation, in which it promotes the degradation of factors V and VIII by activated protein C.

ANTITHROMBIN, α_1-PROTEASE INHIBITOR AND THE SERPINS

STRUCTURE AND FUNCTION

Antithrombin-III and α_1-protease inhibitor belong to the serpin family of plasma glycoprotein inhibitors. While this family includes members such as ovalbumin, which are not protease inhibitors, most inhibit enzymes by formation of a 1:1 covalent complex. This complex forms as a result of covalent bond formation between the active site serine of the enzyme and a specific residue towards the C-terminal end of the serpin, involving cleavage of the backbone of the serpin between two amino acids designated P1 and P1' (Table 6.6). While the resulting complex is stable, a small proportion of the

Table 6.6 Reactive centre sequences of haemostatic serpins

Agent	P4	P3	P2	P1	P1'	P2'	P3'	P4'
α 1-Protease inhibitor	Ala	Ile	Pro	Met	Ser	Ile	Pro	Pro
Antithrombin-III	Ile	Ala	Gly	<u>Arg</u>	Ser	Leu	Asn	Pro
Heparin cofactor II	Phe	Met	Pro	<u>Leu</u>	Ser	Thr	Gln	Val
PAI-1	Val	Ser	Ala	<u>Arg</u>	Met	Ala	Pro	Glu
PAI-2	Met	Thr	Gly	<u>Arg</u>	Thr	Gly	His	Gly
PAI-3/protein C inhibitor	Phe	Thr	Phe	<u>Arg</u>	Ser	Ala	Arg	Leu
Antiplasmin	Ala	Met	Ser	<u>Arg</u>	Met	Ser	Leu	Ser
C1-inhibitor	Ser	Val	Ala	<u>Arg</u>	Thr	Leu	Leu	Val
Protease nexin	Leu	Ile	Ala	<u>Arg</u>	Ser	Ser	Pro	Pro
Recombinant Variants†								
(a) α1-PI: Pittsburgh, Arg-P1	Ala	Ile	Pro	Arg	Ser	Ile	Pro	Pro
(b) α1-PI: AT-III, P1 to P3'	*	*	*	Arg	*	Leu	Asn	*
(c) α1-PI: Ala-P2, Arg-P1	*	*	Ala	Arg	*	Ile	Pro	*
(d) α1-PI: Leu (or Val) P1	*	*	*	Leu	*	*	*	*
(e) α1-PI: Phe-P1	*	*	*	Phe	*	*	*	*
(f) PAI-1: AT-III, P3 to P3'	Val	Ala	Gly	Arg	Ser	Leu	Asn	Glu

†PAI: Plasminogen activator inhibitor.
α1-PI: α 1-protease inhibitor (antitrypsin).
AT-III: Antithrombin-III.
*: Residues as in A1-PI.
Residues underlined form the active site P1 residue of the native serpins and heavily influence the spectrum of enzymes inhibited by the serpin.

product may dissociate releasing active enzyme and cleaved serpin, a reaction promoted by nucleophiles.

The three-dimensional structure of the cleaved form (R-form) of serpins is known from crystallographic studies, but that of the uncleaved type (S-form) is not clear as it has resisted attempts to crystallize it. The recent crystallization of the non-inhibitor serpin ovalbumin suggests that the P1–P1' sequence occurs on an exposed loop of the molecule. Following cleavage of this bond a large conformational change occurs in inhibitors. Unlike the previously discussed coagulent proteins, serpins exhibit no obvious division of the molecule into domains, but are globular proteins of approximately 400 amino acids and molecular weight 50 000.

The specificity of serpins is dependent on the sequence of amino acids around the 'active site' P1 residue. For some of the serpins involved in haemostasis, these sequences are shown in Table 6.6. It will be seen that for many, but by no means all of these, the P1 residue is arginine, which is also the cleavage site residue for many of the substrate pro-enzymes involved in coagulation. Just how critical the P1 residue is, is illustrated by the Pittsburgh variant of antitrypsin in which the P1 methionine is mutated to arginine. This alone changes antitrypsin from an inhibitor primarily directed to elastase, to one with a much-enhanced ability to inhibit thrombin. The patient with this mutation suffered from recurrent bleeds and died young.

Methionine residues in the P1 region of serpins are particularly sensitive to oxidation by laboratory reagents, oxygen radicals or components of tobacco smoke. This is particularly important in the case of α_1-protease inhibitor, whose primary function is to control elastase activity in the lung. In this case, methionine forms the active P1 site and oxidation results in near complete loss of activity. In patients with congenitally low levels of this serpin, smoking can result in inactivating oxidation of the residual inhibitor with loss of protection of the lungs against attack by leukocyte elastase and development of emphysema.

Other areas of the serpin molecules are important for its activity and specificity. Thus in antiplasmin a group of residues in an extended C terminal are involved in binding of this inhibitor to plasmin and plasminogen. This binding occurs very rapidly and with high affinity and is responsible for the remarkable efficiency of antiplasmin in inhibiting plasmin (see Chapter 7). Interestingly binding of vitronectin to PAI-1 reduces its ability to inhibit plasminogen activator but increases thrombin inactivation. This is presumably an indirect effect, but must involve the active site.

The reaction of a number of serpins with their target enzymes is enhanced by the sulphated polysaccharide heparin. This is most dramatic in the case of antithrombin-III which inhibits thrombin, Factor Xa and Factor IXa. Heparin enhances the rates of these reactions by several hundredfold. Hence the use of heparin as a therapeutic anticoagulant. The binding of heparin to antithrombin occurs via a series of positively charged residues in the sides of

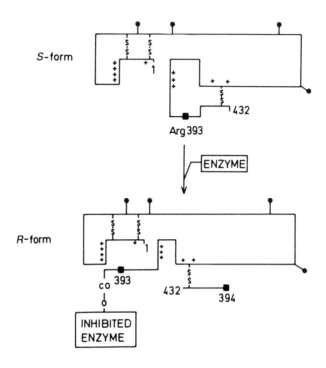

Fig. 6.7. Antithrombin-III structure and function. The 432 amino acid inhibitor contains four carbohydrate chains (————●) and three disulphide bonds (–S–S–). Arginine and lysine residues involved in heparin binding are indicated by + signs. The protein circulates in plasma in a stressed (S) conformation with the reactive site arginine-393 on an exposed surface loop. On reaction with enzyme (e.g. thrombin), an ester bond is formed between the active site serine and the carboxyl group of residue 393. This is accompanied by a large change in conformation to a relaxed (R) form and cleavage of the antithrombin, although the small C-terminal peptide remains attached to the complex through a disulphide bond. A small proportion of the complex may dissociate to active enzyme and inactive, cleaved inhibitor. Similar reactions occur for other serpins during inhibition of serine proteases

a groove on the surface of the molecule. These residues are largely located on the N-terminal half of the molecule. Figure 6.7 illustrates their location in the antithrombin molecule, and also represents the cleavage at arginine-393 occurring during inhibition of thrombin. Similar events occur for other serpins. The affinity of antithrombin for heparin is utilised in the purification of concentrates of this protein from plasma.

DEFICIENCY STATES AND PLASMA-DERIVED CONCENTRATES

The major inhibitor of coagulation is antithrombin-III. Deficiency, as for other serpins, may be quantitative (type I) or qualitative, i.e. due to an inactive molecule (type II). In either case, symptoms of recurrent thrombosis are seen if levels much below 50% of normal activity occur. This is similar to proteins C and S, but unlike Factors VIII and IX deficiency, where severe symptoms are not seen until protein concentrations are < 10% of normal. One result is that most patients diagnosed as antithrombin deficient are heterozygotes and have some normal antithrombin.

Most patients with antithrombin deficiency can be managed using heparin or coumarin anticoagulant therapy, but replacement therapy is useful during pregnancy or to allow major operations. As discussed above, antithrombin concentrate may also be useful in the acquired deficiency seen during disseminated intravascular coagulation. A number of manufacturers prepare a pasteurized antithrombin concentrate prepared by heparin affinity chromatography of plasma.

While α_1-protease has a role in inhibition of protein C, Factors IXa and Xa, the main result of congenital deficiency is susceptibility to lung disease and liver disease. The deficiency state is relatively common, particularly in Anglo-Saxon groups, and most cases are due to occurrence of one of two variants – S or Z – in place of the normal M form. Neither of these involve the active site (methionine-358) of the inhibitor, but do affect formation of internal salt bridges in the molecule with a resultant destabilizing effect. The rarer Z type involves a change from glutamate to lysine at residue 342 disrupting bonding to lysine-290. The more common S type is due to substitution of valine for glutamate-264 which normally interacts with lysine-387. The results of both these changes is to reduce the levels of secreted product. For the Z type this is accompanied by deposition of protein in the liver cells which may explain the occurrence of neonatal hepatitis and liver cancer in later life in some patients. In the S form, liver deposition does not occur and deficiency is presumed to arise from increased intracellular processing of the protein. Each individual receives one gene from each parent. Levels < 50% of normal are seen in individuals with ZZ and SZ forms, but symptoms may also occur in patients with SS and MZ types and plasma levels around 50% of normal. While levels of inhibitor are low in such patients, the protein that is present has inhibitory activity.

The major effect of α_1-protease inhibitor deficiency is a much increased risk of developing lung disease (emphysema). This usually becomes apparent during the third decade of life, particularly in smokers as a result of the inactivation of residual inhibitor by smoke-induced oxidation. At this stage, the loss in lung elasticity caused by the lack of inhibition of elastase is irreversible and any therapy other than a lung transplant, can only halt disease progress, not cure it.

Two pasteurized, plasma-derived concentrates of α_1-protease inhibitor have recently become available. These are prepared by anion-exchange and size-exclusion chromatography of plasma or Cohn fraction IV.I. Both these products are at clinical trial in patients with the deficiency and symptoms of lung dysfunction. Replacement by the intravenous route requires doses of about 4 g each week and is safe. Whether or not it is effective may take some years to establish, but if it does prove effective, current supplies of plasma are unlikely to provide enough material for all patients. In view of this, there has been much interest in recombinant α_1-protease inhibitor or some alternative, such as recombinant secretory leukocyte protease inhibitor – a leukocyte-derived elastase inhibitor. One option is to administer the concentrate as an aerosol directly to where it is needed – the lungs. This has been tried and appears to work and reduces the total dose required by two- to threefold.

RECOMBINANT PRODUCTS

While recombinant antithrombin has been prepared from mammalian cell cultures and shown to be equivalent to the plasma protein, most of the work on therapeutic recombinant serpins has centred on α_1-protease inhibitor. This has been prepared using bacteria, yeast, mammalian cell culture and in transgenic animals. Only the yeast and mammalian culture products have been assessed *in vivo*. Unfortunately, the yeast product is incorrectly glycosylated and is rapidly cleared after intravenous infusion. It may prove useful if intrapulmonary administration is used. High-level expression is feasible from mammalian cell cultures or in the milk of transgenic animals and work on appropriate purification of these products is in hand.

One reason for the interest in recombinant α_1-protease inhibitor is the possibility of changing the inhibitory spectrum of the molecule by minor changes in the active site region. The Pittsburgh variant (Met-358 to Arg) which results in conversion from an elastase to thrombin inhibitor has been mentioned. Recombinant versions of this natural variant have been produced. Heparin does not influence the rate of inhibition of thrombin by this variant and it inhibits thrombin faster than antithrombin in the absence of heparin. This variant also inhibits Factor XIIa and kallikrein more than the parent molecule.

Illustrative examples of other recombinant variants of the active site region of serpins are given in Table 6.6. Substitution of leucine or valine at P1 (Table 6.6, d) gives a product which is still a cathepsin and elastase inhibitor but resists oxidation, as it no longer contains the susceptible methionine. Substitution of phenylalanine at this position (e) gives a specific inhibitor of leukocyte cathepsin D. With a P2 alanine as well as arginine P1 (c), the protein has enhanced reactivity with kallikrein. In contrast, if the P1 to P3' sequence of α_1-protease inhibitor is replaced by that from antithrombin (b), the ability to inhibit cathepsin is reduced but inhibition of plasmin, elastase and trypsin is retained or enhanced. A similar substitution of antithrombin sequence into PAI-1 (f) increases thrombin inhibition at the expense of inhibition of plasminogen activators. These studies suggest the feasibility of tailoring the inhibitor of choice by a 'pick-and-mix' process using natural sequences.

All these changes involve the active site region of serpins. The potential for tailoring other parts of the molecule has yet to be fully explored. One could consider, for example, incorporation of the antiplasmin C-terminal regional to localize inhibitor to plasminogen.

OTHER INHIBITORS

The serpin C-1-esterase inhibitor can inhibit Factors XIIa and XIa but the requirement for these factors in normal coagulation is uncertain. A more important consequence of C-1-inhibitor deficiency is the occurrence of an-gioneurotic oedema. This can be treated with replacement therapy during acute attacks and plasma-derived concentrates of this protein are available. Recombinant serpins which inhibit the appropriate reactions have been developed.

α_2-Macroglobulin acts as a reserve inhibitor of many haemostatic enzymes if the primary inhibitor is depleted. Severe deficiency has not been described and may be fatal. Neither plasma-derived or recombinant concentrate is available.

Both high-molecular-weight kininogen, which is involved in the activation of Factor XIa, and histidine-rich glycoprotein (see Chapter 7) contain regions similar to those found in cystatins. These are inhibitors of enzymes with a cysteine active site, such as calpain or pepsin. While such enzymes are not directly involved in coagulation they are involved, for example, in the activation of platelets. The inhibitors may thus have an indirect influence on haemostasis.

The extrinsic path inhibitor (EPI) is a plasma glycoprotein of about 40000 Da with a negatively charged N-terminal and a positively charged C-terminal. On binding to Factor Xa, the complex is able to reversibly inhibit the tissue factor–VIIa complex. The EPI molecule contains three Kunitz inhibitor domains, which are also found in certain plant enzyme inhibitors and plasma inter-α-trypsin inhibitor. The first two of these domains are necessary for the binding of EPI to Factors VIIa and Xa, respectively. The function of the third domain is unknown but could involve interactions with lipoproteins for which EPI exhibits a strong association. Using a recombinant approach, a chimaeric molecule consisting of the light chain of Factor Xa and the first Kunitz domain of EPI in one molecule has been prepared. This protein is able to inhibit tissue Factor VIIa in the absence of Factor Xa and may prove useful in therapy of unwanted coagulation caused by the release or exposure of tissue factor in patients.

FURTHER READING

Carrell, R. and Travis, J. (1985) Alpha-1-antitrypsin and the serpins: Variation and countervariation. *Trends in Biochemical Sciences*, **10**, 20–24.

Dolan, G., Ball, J. and Preston, F.E. (1989) Protein C and protein S. *Baillière's Clinical Haematology*, **2**, 999–1042.

Gadek, J.E. (1988) Alpha-1-antitrypsin deficiency. Usage of alpha-1-proteinase inhibitor concentrate in replacement therapy. *American Journal of Medicine*, **84**(6A), 1–90.

Gianelli, F. (1989) Factor IX. *Baillière's Clinical Haematology*, **2**, 821–848.

Kane, W.H. and Davie, E.W. (1988) Blood coagulation Factor V and VIII: Structural and functional similarities and their relationship to hemorrhagic and thrombotic disorders. *Blood*, **71**, 539–555.

Mann, K.G., Nesheim, M.E., Church, W.E., Haley, P. and Krishnaswarmy, S. (1990) Surface dependent reactions of the vitamin K-dependent enzyme complexes. *Blood*, **76**, 1–16.

Manson, H.E., Austin, R.C., Fernandez-Rachubinski, F., Rachubinski, R.A. and Blajchman, M.A. (1989) The molecular pathology of inherited antithrombin-III deficiency. *Transfusion Medicine Review*, **III**, 264–281.

Meulien, P. and Tuddenham, E.G.D. (1990) Genetically engineered and affinity purified plasma proteins. *Baillière's Clinical Haematology*, **3**, 451–477.

Simons, J.P., Wilmut, I., Clarke, A.J., Archibald, A.L., Bishop, J.O. and Lathe, R. (1988) Gene transfer in sheep. *Biotechnology*, **6**, 179–183.

Titani, K. and Walsh, K.A. (1988) Human von Willebrand factor: The molecular glue of platelet plugs. *Trends in Biochemical Sciences*, **13**, 94–97.

7 Fibrinolysis

I.R. MacGREGOR and N.A. BOOTH

MECHANISMS OF FIBRINOLYSIS

Fibrinolysis is the process responsible for dissolving the fibrin matrix of thrombi and injured tissues. The system centres on the activation of plasminogen to form plasmin, the protease that lyses fibrin (Figure 7.1). There are two human enzymes that carry out this reaction, t-PA (tissue plasminogen activator) and u-PA (urokinase). The plasminogen activators and plasmin are all serine proteases. The active proteases are inhibited by specific inhibitors. The main plasminogen activator inhibitors are PAI-1 and PAI-2. Plasmin is inhibited principally by α_2-antiplasmin (α_2-AP). Like their target proteases, these inhibitors are structurally and functionally related.

A common feature of the serine proteases is that the active enzyme arises by cleavage of a single-chain precursor or zymogen. The two chains of the protease are held together by disulphide bonds. The active site of all the serine proteases is located in the B (light) chain, while the A (heavy) chain contains structural domains that have important binding properties. These domains are each encoded by distinct exons, which is significant for the evolution of this protein family. Some general features of plasmin, t-PA and u-PA, the three principal enzymes of fibrinolysis are summarized in Figure 7.2.

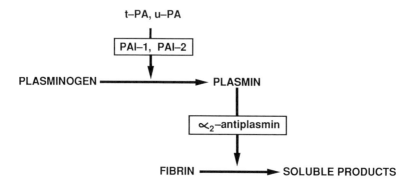

Fig. 7.1. Pathway of fibrinolysis

Plasma and Recombinant Blood Products in Medical Therapy
Edited by C.V. Prowse. Published 1992 by John Wiley & Sons Ltd

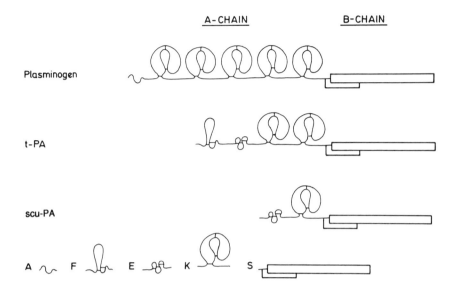

Fig. 7.2. Domains common to plasminogen, t-PA, u-PA. K = kringle (lysine-binding region); E = epidermal growth factor-like region; F = fibronectin finger-like fibrin-binding region; S = serine protease (active site); A = activation peptide.

PLASMINOGEN

Plasminogen is a single-chain 92 kDa glycoprotein. The A chain contains five homologous regions, known as 'kringles'. These domains contain lysine-binding sites, which interact with lysine and its analogues, 6-aminocaproic acid and tranexamic acid. The kringle 1 lysine-binding site has the highest affinity for lysine (K_d 9 μM), while those of kringles 2–5 have lower affinity (K_d 5 mM). The lysine-binding sites are responsible for the binding of plasminogen (and plasmin) to fibrin, a crucially-important property for the regulation of fibrinolysis. Interactions between plasmin and its principal inhibitor, α_2-antiplasmin, also involve these sites.

Plasminogen circulates at a relatively high concentration (2 μM) and it has a plasma half-life of about 2 days. A significant proportion of plasma plasminogen is normally bound to histidine-rich glycoprotein, which reduces the concentration of plasminogen available for potential activation to about 1 μM. The lysine-binding sites of plasminogen are involved in this interaction.

t-PA (TISSUE PLASMINOGEN ACTIVATOR)

Tissue plasminogen activator is a glycoprotein of about 65 kDa. It is an unusual serine protease in that it has considerable activity in its single-chain form. The A chain domains of t-PA include a finger region, a growth factor domain and two kringles that are homologous to those of plasminogen.

T-PA binds strongly to fibrin via its finger region and its second kringle. Further, the activity of t-PA is fibrin specific. The activation of plasminogen by t-PA is relatively inefficient in the absence of fibrin but greatly enhanced in its presence. This is due to an increased affinity of t-PA for plasminogen when fibrin is present. These properties of t-PA are central to the regulation of fibrinolysis and to its use as a therapeutic thrombolytic agent.

The normal plasma concentration of t-PA is low (about 5 ng/ml) but it rises in response to physiological and pharmacological stimuli, including exercise, venous occlusion and vasopressin analogues.

u-PA (UROKINASE)

This plasminogen activator cleaves the same bond in plasminogen as does t-PA but, in marked contrast to t-PA, u-PA cleaves plasminogen efficiently in the absence of fibrin. The single-chain form of u-PA (scu-PA) is relatively inactive but can be activated to the two-chain form (tcu-PA) by plasmin or by kallikrein. The A chain contains two domains that are similar to those in t-PA. These are a growth factor domain and a kringle. The absence of a finger domain and of the second kringle explains why u-PA (either sc or tc) does not bind to fibrin.

For many years t-PA was regarded as the only important activator in the circulation. It is now clear that u-PA occurs also in the circulation, primarily in its single-chain form, at a plasma concentration of about 2 ng/ml. Its physiological and pathological role in the circulation is not yet well defined.

STREPTOKINASE

This is not a human protein but is included since it is widely used as a therapeutic agent. Streptokinase (SK), a product of some streptococcal strains, has no enzymatic activity but it forms a fibrinolytically active complex with plasminogen.

α_2-ANTIPLASMIN

This glycoprotein of apparent molecular mass 70 kDa is the major inhibitor of plasmin. It reacts very rapidly with plasmin; the rate constant for their reaction is 2×10^7 M^{-1}s^{-1}. This fast reaction, coupled with the relatively high plasma concentration of α_2-antiplasmin (about 1 μM) makes this inhibitor an important element in the regulation of fibrinolysis.

PLASMINOGEN ACTIVATOR INHIBITORS

PAI-1

PAI-1 is a glycoprotein of about 48 kDa and it occurs in plasma and platelets and in a number of cultured cells, notably endothelial cells. PAI-1 is a very potent inhibitor of t-PA and u-PA, with a rate constant of 10^7 $M^{-1}s^{-1}$, comparable to that for α_2-antiplasmin-plasmin (Table 7.1). Unlike α_2-antiplasmin, its plasma concentration is low, about 20 ng/ml. PAI-1 is an acute-phase reactant and its plasma concentration is high in several diseases. Elevated PAI-1 is thought to be associated with increased risk of thromboembolic disease.

Platelets represent an important pool of PAI-1, independent of plasma PAI-1, and accounting for > 90% of the circulating inhibitor. Plasma and platelet PAI-1 differ in activity. PAI-1 can occur in an inactive (latent) form that can be activated under denaturing conditions. While plasma PAI-1 is almost all active, platelet PAI-1 is only 3–5% active but can be reactivated following denaturation. Whether there are physiological conditions under which such activation occurs is not yet understood. It should be noted that platelets still account for about half the circulating PAI-1 activity, the relatively poor activity of this PAI-1 being compensated for by its high concentration.

PAI-2

PAI-2 is immunologically distinct from PAI-1 but has similar specificity. It has a lower affinity than PAI-1 for both t-PA and u-PA. It is notable that it is a very poor inhibitor of single-chain t-PA. It occurs in placenta, in pregnancy plasma and is thought to be primarily a placental protein that functions in securing haemostasis at the placento-uterine interface. It occurs also in peripheral blood monocytes and in related cultured cells (e.g. U937) and may have a more general role in non-pregnant individuals.

PAI-3

This inhibitor was discovered in urine and it occurs also in plasma. It is now known to be primarily an inhibitor of activated protein C. At its normal plasma concentration of about 2 µg/ml, it is unlikely to contribute to physiological inhibition of t-PA and u-PA (Table 7.1).

Table 7.1 Inhibitors of fibrinolysis

Inhibitor	Rate constants $(M^{-1}s^{-1})$			
	α_2-AP	PAI-1	PAI-2	PAI-3
sct-PA		10^7	9×10^2	$<10^3$
tct-PA		$>10^7$	2×10^5	$<10^3$
tcu-PA		$>10^7$	10^6	8×10^3
Plasmin	3×10^7			10^2
Plasma concentration	70µg/ml (1µM)	20ng/ml (0.4nM)	0*	2µg/ml (40nM)

* Late pregnancy plasma concentration 250 ng/ml (4 nM).

REGULATION OF FIBRINOLYSIS

Fibrinolysis, like all serine protease cascade systems, is regulated by the activation of zymogens to active enzymes and the specific inhibition of the active enzymes, as well as by the concentrations of these proteins in the circulation. Over and above these general mechanisms, fibrin has a central regulatory role. Both plasminogen and t-PA bind strongly to fibrin, so that plasmin can be produced at its site of action. Further, activation of plasminogen by t-PA occurs very much more efficiently on the fibrin surface than in the absence of fibrin. Plasminogen in the circulation is not normally activated to form plasmin; activation occurs preferentially on the fibrin surface.

The regulatory mechanism is further enhanced by the effects of the major plasmin inhibitor, α_2-antiplasmin. This is avid in sequestering any plasmin formed in the circulation, which has a half-life of only about 100 ms. Plasmin formed on the fibrin surface is relatively protected from the action of its inhibitor. Not only is its active site occupied by its substrate, fibrin, but its lysine-binding sites are also occupied by fibrin. Thus its capacity to interact with α_2-antiplasmin is greatly diminished.

This explanation for the regulation of plasminogen by t-PA also explains the fact that, although u-PA does not bind to fibrin, its single-chain form does promote fibrin-specific lysis. Plasmin activates scu-PA to form tcu-PA. Since plasmin is protected on the fibrin surface, it follows that the activation of scu-PA will occur there.

PURIFICATION OF FIBRINOLYTIC PROTEINS

PLASMINOGEN FROM PLASMA

Lysine-Sepharose is used as an affinity gel for the large-scale production of plasminogen. The lysine groups bind to the plasminogen lysine-binding sites in the kringle structures, thereby immobilizing plasminogen on the gel matrix. Batches of plasma up to 2500 litres are used. Plasma is first depleted of fibrinogen and cold insoluble globulin by cold ethanol fractionation (Cohn's method). The plasminogen-containing supernatant is then mixed batchwise with lysine-Sepharose. After washing the gel, slurry is packed into a chromatographic column which is washed with a buffer of increasing ionic strength. This elutes unwanted proteins bound to the gel by non-specific ionic interactions. Plasminogen is then eluted by displacing it from the lysine-Sepharose with a buffer containing lysine or ε-aminocaproic acid.

α_2-ANTIPLASMIN FROM PLASMA

α_2-antiplasmin is most readily purified from a cold ethanol fraction of plasma that is depleted of plasminogen, thereby permitting an affinity chromatography step using plasminogen-Sepharose. Subsequent ion-exchange chromatography with DEAE-Sephadex and affinity chromatography with concanavalin A lectin-Sepharose results in a product of high purity.

t-PA MADE FROM TISSUE-CULTURE SOURCES

The plasma concentration of t-PA is inadequate as a source for purification. A clinical dose of 100 mg t-PA would require about 10 000 litres of plasma starting material! Tissue extracts such as human placenta and porcine hearts have been used as sources of t-PA for extraction and purification. A t-PA product derived from eluates of human cadaver blood vessels has been used clinically in the Soviet Union for a number of years. None of these sources yields the predicted amounts of t-PA needed for wider clinical use.

Various transformed human cell lines have been used as sources of t-PA for purification, and initial animal studies and clinical trials utilized such material. The human Bowes melanoma cell line typically secretes 0.5 mg t-PA per litre of culture supernatant, and is readily grown as bulk cultures. Unlike non-transformed cell lines, the melanoma line can be repeatedly sub-cultured. Because the culture medium is devoid of serum, the secreted t-PA represents a relatively high proportion (ca. 0.5%) of total protein in the medium. This simplifies purification procedures, which have usually used affinity techniques.

Immobilized metal-ion affinity chromatography is employed as a concentration/purifying step, by binding histidine residues present on t-PA. A protein of acceptably high purity is then obtained by subsequent use of the immobilized lectin concanavalin A which binds to carbohydrate side-chains on t-PA, and gel-filtration chromatography which removes unwanted high-molecular-weight aggregates of t-PA and permits equilibration of the purified t-PA in a suitable buffer.

A second approach uses monoclonal antibodies against t-PA, immobilized to Sepharose. The resulting enzyme–antibody complex can be dissociated by chaotropes such as potassium thiocyanate or by changes in buffer pH, after washing away non-specifically bound contaminating proteins in a buffer of high ionic strength. Such immunoaffinity purified t-PA can be obtained with high yield and purity. Contamination of the product with mouse immunoglobulins leached from the immunoaffinity support is minimized by suitable column washing steps allied to assay for mouse proteins in the final product.

The hydrophobic nature of t-PA requires the addition of non-ionic detergents to all buffers to reduce losses through adsorption and aggregation. In addition the broadly-specific protease inhibitor aprotinin may be used to reduce proteolytic conversion of one-chain to two-chain t-PA.

If a single therapeutic dose of t-PA is taken as 100 mg (as an approximation) then about 100 litres of medium conditioned by t-PA secreting cells will

Table 7.2 Molecular cloning

Protein	mRNA (kb)	Protein amino acids (number of amino acids)	Structural domains*
Plasmin (ogen)	2.9	790	5-K; S
t-PA	2.7	530	E; F; 2-K; S
u-PA	2.4	411	E; K; S
α₂-antiplasmin	2.2	452	PI
PAI-1	3.0	379	PI

* Key: K = kringle lysine-binding region; E = epidermal growth factor-like region; F = fibronectin finger-like fibrin-binding region; S = serine protease (active site); PI = serine protease inhibitor reactive centre.

be needed to provide this amount. Clearly extremely large cell 'factories' are needed to achieve such output. Enhanced secretion of t-PA has been achieved by introducing extra copies of the human t-PA gene into this cell line.

t-PA MADE FROM RECOMBINANT DNA SOURCES

Because of the limitation on the amount of native t-PA secreted by transformed cell lines, t-PA production based on recombinant DNA technology has been developed. Table 7.2 lists some of the genomic properties of fibrinolytic enzymes and inhibitors.

E. coli as host

Products in bacterial hosts may be secreted, stored as soluble intracellular material or as insoluble aggregates. The desired route can be selected during the gene-cloning process. Although recombinant t-PA (rt-PA) can be extracted from aggregates and resolubilized with correct refolding of the protein chain, correct attachment of carbohydrate side-chains (glycosylation) cannot occur. *Bacillus subtilis* is also used as a host where t-PA is recovered in an inactive form in intracellular inclusion bodies. Activation is achieved by complete reduction of the t-PA followed by slow oxidation.

Yeast as host

Active human t-PA has been expressed in, and purified from, yeast cells. Since secretion of yeast proteins can be maintained at very low levels the secreted t-PA represents a high proportion of total protein thereby simplifying subsequent purification stages. Glycosylation with the correct oligosaccharides, which comprise about 12% of the t-PA molecule by weight, does not occur. This appears to be unimportant for the full expression of biological activity although some effects upon clearance rate after injection may be observed.

Mammalian cells as host

Using mammalian cells as host, it is possible to obtain correct glycosylation, disulphide bridge formation and other post-translational modifications that lead to correct ternary protein structure. Chinese hamster ovary (CHO) cells are used successfully for t-PA production, while mouse and other cell lines have also been evaluated. Drawbacks with mammalian cells relate to their lower cell densities compared with microorganisms, high costs of growth medium, presence of pathogens and oncogenes, and difficulty in maintaining viability. Despite these factors, mammalian cells are the host system of choice for large complex proteins such as t-PA, which require extensive post-translational modifications.

u-PA/scu-PA MADE FROM RECOMBINANT DNA SOURCES

scu-PA has been purified after expression in mouse, hamster and human (embryonic kidney) cell-line host systems. The higher degrees of glycosylation seen in these recombinant proteins compared with native scu-PA purified from human urine does not influence the conversion to two-chain u-PA catalysed by plasmin, nor the activity of the two-chain form in cleaving plasminogen. All forms are equally susceptible to inhibition by PAI-1.

A recombinant low-molecular-weight derivative of scu-PA, containing only amino acids 144–411, has been expressed in high yield in CHO cells. Its fibrinolytic properties are identical with intact scu-PA and illustrate how an engineering approach can lead to efficient production of a protein devoid of redundant sequences.

PLASMINOGEN MADE FROM RECOMBINANT DNA SOURCES

Attempts to express plasminogen in mammalian cell lines have resulted in secretion of degraded forms of the molecule. This is not unexpected in view of the ubiquitous distribution of plasminogen activators in such cells and so a host has been sought that is devoid of plasminogen activators. Since invertebrate cell lines fulfil such criteria, a recombinant human plasminogen has been expressed in an insect cell line. It has a molecular weight similar to native plasma glu-plasminogen, binds to lysine-Sepharose and is activated to plasmin by urokinase. Interactions with polyclonal and monoclonal antibodies directed against various epitopes (binding sites) on plasma plasminogen indicate that the expressed molecule has undergone post-translational modifications that result in correct refolding of the single polypeptide chain. This source of plasminogen could supplement plasma-derived material used in thrombolytic therapy if sufficiently high expression can be achieved.

PAI-1 MADE FROM TISSUE CULTURE AND RECOMBINANT DNA SOURCES

Present at only microgram per litre concentrations in plasma, this serine protease inhibitor has been purified from endothelial, HT 1080 fibrosarcoma, Hep G2 hepatoma and MJZJ melanoma cells, which secrete at milligram per litre amounts. PAI-1 is an ideal candidate for production by recombinant DNA methods to yield the amounts of material needed for biochemical and pharmacological studies, because it contains no cysteine residues and therefore no intra-chain disulphide bridges. Thus the potential problem of incorrect disulphide bridging leading to wrong folding does not exist.

Escherichia coli

Human recombinant PAI-1 purified from lysates of transformed *E. coli* cells, yields an unglycosylated active PAI-1 with a molecular weight of 43 kDa.

Yeast

PAI-1 produced intracellularly in *Saccharomyces cerevisiae* yields 8 mg human PAI-1 per litre of confluent yeast culture. The recombinant PAI-1, purified at a recovery of 20%, exhibits properties similar to native PAI-1 with regard to kinetics of inactivation of t-PA and to conversion between latent and active forms. These similarities argue against a role for carbohydrate moieties on PAI-1 in these properties of the molecule, since the above protein is synthesized in an unglycosylated form.

CHO cells

Recombinant human PAI-1 secreted by transfected CHO cells at 1mg/litre conditioned medium has physio-chemical and functional properties similar to native PAI-1.

OTHER PAIs AND ANTIPLASMIN

A PAI has been purified from the histiocytic lymphoma cell line U-937 at yields of 20 mg/litre conditioned medium, and is immunologically identical to the PAI designated PAI-2 derived from human placenta.

   Recombinant human monocyte cell line-derived PAI-2 has been expressed in *E. coli* as an unglycosylated protein of 46.5 kDa. It reacts with urokinase to form an enzymatically inactive complex. Experiments utilizing a rabbit reticulocyte expression system indicate that PAI-2 shares an unusual property with chicken ovalbumin (its nearest serine protease inhibitor family homologue) of being glycosylated and secreted efficiently without the prior cleavage of a signal peptide.

Recombinant human α_2-antiplasmin has been expressed in a Baby Hamster Kidney (BHK) cell line. The molecular mass of the secreted protein (omitting the contribution of the propeptide sequence) at 67 kDa is indistinguishable from that of native human plasma α_{-2}-antiplasmin. Affinity for plasmin(ogen) and inhibitory activity towards plasmin is identical to native inhibitor. However, ability to form crosslinks with fibrin is diminished, probably due to steric hindrance of the α_2-antiplasmin–fibrin binding site caused by the retained propeptide at the amino terminus region.

CLINICAL APPLICATIONS

REPLACEMENT THERAPY

Plasminogen has been used occasionally to supplement circulating plasma levels in patients with inherited deficiencies where thrombotic tendencies are seen. Such deficiency states are rare, probably because the defect is life-threatening at an early stage of development. Likewise α_2-antiplasmin has been used infrequently to treat bleeding complications associated with a deficiency of this fibrinolytic inhibitor.

LYSIS OF BLOOD CLOTS

Uses of plasminogen

The main use of plasminogen is in treatments designed to lyse blood clots, usually referred to as 'thrombolytic therapy'. Streptokinase, derived from haemolytic streptococci, has been used as a thrombolytic agent since the 1950s. Unlike t-PA or u-PA, it is inherently proteolytically inactive but forms an enzymatically active complex with plasminogen that can convert free plasminogen to plasmin. While streptokinase is usually injected alone, a preformed streptokinase–plasminogen complex (streptodornase) is also used clinically, with the aim of maintaining plasminogen levels and thereby promoting further plasminogen-to-plasmin conversion.

After myocardial infarction, streptokinase has been found to reduce mortality during hospitalization from 11.7 to 8.9%, in a trial of 17 189 patients randomly allocated to receive streptokinase, oral aspirin, both or neither (ISIS-2 study). However, the high incidence of bleeding associated with this therapy, including a 1–3% reported incidence of cerebral haemorrhage, has certainly limited its wider use.

A successful approach to limit such side-effects has been developed in Beecham's acylated plasminogen streptokinase complex (APSAC). Here the

Table 7.3 Properties of current thrombolytic agents

Agent	SK	APSAC	u-PA	scu-PA	t-PA
Degrades circulating fibrinogen*	+++	++	+++	+	+
Antigenic	Yes	Yes	No	No	No
Circulating antibodies may reduce response	Yes	Yes	No	No	No
Natural inhibitors	No	No	Yes	Yes	Yes
Bleeding problems	Yes	Yes	Yes	Yes††	Yes††
Mode of injection†	I	BI	I	I	I

* +, ++, +++ indicate increasing levels of fibrinogen degradation observed during therapeutic use.
† I = infusion; BI = bolus injection.
†† While they have been observed, bleeding problems associated with the use of the scu-PA and t-PA are less obvious than for the other three agents.

active centre responsible for converting plasminogen to plasmin is blocked by acylation with a *p*-anisolyl derivative. *In vivo*, this site becomes available after injection by slow deacylation. This results in a prolonged thrombolytic effect without exceedingly high initial plasmin generation, with the advantage that the drug can be given by bolus rather than slow infusion. This raises the possibility of it being administered by general practitioners or paramedics prior to hospitalization of the patient and the value of early thrombolytic treatment in myocardial infarction is well known.

Comparison of currently available thrombolytic agents

Thrombosis and embolism are major causes of death and disability in cardiovascular diseases and thrombolytic therapy has applications in myocardial infarction, cerebrovascular thrombosis and venous thromboembolism. Thrombolytic therapy has been used occasionally to treat deep venous thrombosis and combined with heparin it is a treatment of choice in some types of major acute pulmonary embolism. Occlusion of peripheral arteries may be cleared by local infusion of thrombolytic agents. The hazards may outweigh the benefits of thrombolysis in major ischaemic stroke and such therapy is still at an early stage of development. This leaves acute myocardial infarction which is the most common indication for thrombolytic therapy. The main properties of currently used agents are shown in Tables 7.3 and 7.4.

Large clinical trials have demonstrated that streptokinase and t-PA are effective at inducing reperfusion and patency in an occluded coronary vessel. Smaller trials indicate that APSAC, u-PA and scu-PA are also efficient thrombolytic agents. Reperfusion is achieved in about 43% of patients infused with streptokinase and 70% where t-PA is used. Likewise vessel patency is seen in 50% and 75% of patients receiving streptokinase and t-PA, respectively. This is reflected in a reduction in early mortality of at least 25%.

Table 7.4 Therapeutic doses of thrombolytic agents in current wide use

Thrombolytic agent	Trade name	Dosage	Duration of infusion (min)
Streptokinase	Kabikinase Streptase	1.5×10^6 U (= 15 mg)	60
APSAC	Eminase	30 mg	5
Urokinase	Abbokinase Actosolv Ukidan Persolv	3×10^6 U (= 30 mg)	30–60
t-PA	Activase	100 mg	180

The main side-effect of thrombolytic therapy is bleeding and strokes. Although bleeding is less likely with t-PA then streptokinase, it is still a common problem. This is due to the inability of t-PA to distinguish between fibrin in an occluding thrombus and fibrin forming a haemostatic plug, for example at the site of arterial catheterization. Since re-occlusion of the coronary vessel can re-occur, heparin is often given in the later stages of thrombolytic therapy with t-PA, which may worsen the risk of bleeding.

Secondary properties of thrombolytic agents are particularly likely to influence their perceived usefulness, at least until further larger trials with the newer agents are finished. Streptokinase is currently (1991) the cheapest at about £120 per dose compared with about £1000 for a dose of t-PA and £400 for APSAC. But streptokinase induces antibodies that limit its repeated use. Although APSAC has the same drawback, it is unique in the ability to inject it as a bolus rather than slow infusion, as described above. t-PA possesses an affinity for fibrin that reduces bleeding complications and is non-antigenic.

IMPROVING ON NATURE

ENGINEERED t-PA FOR RESISTANCE TO PAI

PAI-1 inhibits t-PA by binding to its active site and thereby preventing it from binding plasminogen and converting it to plasmin. Studies on the trypsin–trypsin inhibitor system have shown that inhibitor may interact with its target enzyme at sites other than the reactive centre. On the basis of these data, site-directed mutations in t-PA have been directed to amino acids important for binding to PAI-1 but unimportant for interaction with plasminogen. One such mutant t-PA is inhibited by PAI-1 at 1/20th the rate of native t-PA, and is also less susceptible to inhibition by other plasma protease inhibitors. Such mutant proteins have the potential of retaining activity in environments where inhibitor activity is high, for example at the site of a platelet-rich clot.

ENGINEERED t-PA FOR LONGER HALF-LIFE

Because t-PA is cleared with a half-life of only a few minutes, efforts have been made to prolong the therapeutic effect by modifying regions in t-PA responsible for binding to clearance receptors.

The N-terminus region of t-PA contains a domain with similarities to the fibrin binding finger region of fibronectin (Figure 7.2). Substitutions or deletions of amino acids within the fibronectin finger-like domain of t-PA have been evaluated for their effects upon fibrinolytic activity of t-PA and rate of clearance from the circulation. t-PA variants tend to exhibit reduced *in vitro* fibrinolytic activity. However, a region of the finger domain has been identified in which substitutions can result in variants that are cleared up to sixfold more slowly than native t-PA while retaining fibrinolytic activity. Thus a variant with the changes Gln-42→Asn, His-44→Glu, Asn-117→Gln is fourfold more potent than native t-PA in lysing venous clots in rabbits.

The kringle 2 region of t-PA has been expressed in *E. coli* and utilized for NMR spectroscopy. Marked similarities with plasminogen kringle 4 indicate a likely role in fibrin binding. Studies with deletion mutants of the heavy chain of t-PA indicate that while both finger and kringle 2 domains are important for fibrin binding, only the latter exhibits enhanced binding dependent upon plasmin-mediated generation of carboxyl terminal lysine residues in fibrin.

A simplified t-PA has been expressed in a Syrian hamster cell line, where amino acid residues 4–175 were deleted from the full-length sequence of t-PA. These residues encompass the epidermal growth factor and fibronectin finger domains as well as kringle 1. Delayed clearance of this modified t-PA in dogs, at 20-fold the half-life of native t-PA, is accompanied by apparently better clot dissolution in occluded canine coronary arteries.

A further way in which clearance rate of t-PA can be modified is by removal of a mannose glycosylation site that interacts with liver mannose clearance receptors. This has been achieved by substituting the amino acid asparagine, which forms the glycosylation site, by glutamine which cannot be glycosylated. The mutant t-PA so produced has a threefold slower rate of clearance, confirming the role of this carbohydrate linkage region in clearance mechanisms.

ENGINEERED u-PA FOR RESISTANCE TO PROTEOLYTIC DEGRADATION

scu-PA is converted to an active plasminogen activator (tcu-PA) with fibrin selectivity by limited proteolytic cleavage by plasmin. If plasmin activity is unchecked the active tcu-PA is degraded to a less active low-molecular-weight form. By engineering a variant with less susceptibility to the secondary cleavage by plasmin and thrombin it has been possible to produce a molecule with a greater potential resistance to degradation *in vivo*.

HYBRID AND CHIMAERIC PAs

Hybrid molecules contain regions from two or more proteins fused together. Chimaeric molecules additionally contain one or more amino acid residues altered from the parent molecules. The objective in producing such proteins is to obtain a molecule combining desired characteristics derived from its different component parts.

Hybrids of t-PA and u-PA have been constructed using recombinant DNA technology. A hybrid of t-PA heavy chain that contains the fibrin binding regions responsible for providing the fibrin specificity of this thrombolytic agent was fused with the light chain of u-PA that contains the catalytic, enzymatically active, region. Increased fibrin binding compared with u-PA is observed. However, fusion of t-PA kringle or finger domains, each of which confers part of the fibrin binding activity, with u-PA light chain, results in no increase in fibrin binding.

Similar results have been obtained with a scu-PA in which t-PA kringle 2 was inserted remote from the active site region. Further, addition of another kringle 2 to the double kringle structure in t-PA decreases fibrin-dependent plasminogen activation. Such data indicate that structural domains within a serine protease polypeptide chain may not refold and/or function independently of each other. They therefore impose constraints upon the type of hybrid molecules that can be effectively constructed.

TARGETING OF SUBSTRATE

None of the present generation of thrombolytic agents is absolutely specific for fibrin in a thrombus with the result that degradation of systemic fibrinogen or fibrin in the haemostatic clot can lead to bleeding problems. Attempts have been made to link plasminogen activators to molecules with high specificity for fibrin or other components of clots such as activated platelets, and thereby improve their effectiveness.

Monoclonal antibodies can be raised to neoantigens on fibrin, i.e. to sites that are not exposed in circulating fibrinogen but are present in a fibrin clot. One such successful approach has chemically linked the antigen-binding fragment of a monoclonal antibody with high affinity for crosslinked fibrin, present in a formed thrombus, to the abbreviated form of scu-PA described above. The fibrin specificity of this chimaeric protein is several times higher than for the scu-PA alone.

The success of the above approach has led to attempts to produce the chimaeric antibody-activator protein by recombinant DNA methods. The antibody heavy chain contains the antigen binding region and the gene for this part of the molecule has been cloned, and combined in an expression vector with the sequence coding for the plasminogen activator. The expressed protein (construct) retains the fibrin specificity of the antibody and the fibrinolytic activity of the plasminogen activator.

FURTHER READING

Collen, D.C. and Gold, H.K. (1990) New developments in thrombolytic therapy. *Thrombosis Research,* Suppl. X, 105–131.

Collen, D., Lijnen, H.R., Todd, P.A. and Goa, K.L. (1989) Tissue-type plasminogen activator. A review of its pharmacology and therapeutic use as a thrombolytic agent. *Drugs,* **28**, 346–388.

Haber, E., Quertermous, T., Matsueda, G.R. and Runge, M.S. (1989) Innovative approaches to plasminogen activator therapy. *Science,* **243**, 51–56.

Loskutoff, D.J., Sawdey, M. and Mimuro, J. (1989) Type 1 plasminogen activator inhibitor. *Progress in Hemostasis and Thrombosis,* **9**, 87–115.

Pannekoek, H., de Vries, C. and van Zonneveld, A-J. (1988) Mutants of human tissue-type plasminogen activator (t-PA): structural aspects and functional properties. *Fibrinolysis,* **2**, 123–132.

8 Therapeutic Antibodies

M.C. McCANN and J.E. BOYD

INTRODUCTION

The beneficial effects of antibodies in passive immunotherapy for the prevention and treatment of infectious diseases have long been appreciated. Previously, animal antisera were used in the treatment of diphtheria. However, it was found that repeated administration of foreign protein (e.g. immune horse serum) resulted in 'serum sickness', a complication which arose due to the systemic immune response evoked by repeated exposure to horse serum proteins. These complications led to their replacement by immune human plasma-derived products (Table 8.1).

Table 8.1 Plasma-derived therapeutic immunoglobulin preparations in current use

Anti-tetanus toxoid	Anti-Rhesus (D)
Anti-hepatitis B	Anti-rubella
Anti-rabies	Anti-measles
Anti-hepatitis A	Anti-herpes zoster
Anti-cytomegalovirus	

The plasma required for the preparation of such products is usually obtained by screening the normal blood donor panel and then recruiting those donors with high levels of relevant antibodies (e.g. anti-tetanus; anti-cytomegalovirus) for plasma donation. Despite the improved safety of human plasma-derived therapeutic preparations, there are a number of disadvantages in the use of plasma as a source of specific antibody for therapy.

- *Availability*
  Limited volume
  Restricted range of antigenic specificities
- *Potency*
  Inability to immunize or boost donors in order to manipulate the potency of the material obtained

Plasma and Recombinant Blood Products in Medical Therapy
Edited by C.V. Prowse.   Published 1992 by John Wiley & Sons Ltd

- *Biological efficacy*
  Antibody obtained of restricted immunoglobulin class
  Therapeutic preparation obtained may be unable to effect the required biological function (e.g. phagocytosis, complement fixation, antibody-dependent cell-mediated cytotoxicity (ADCC))
- *Safety*
  The risk of transmission of blood-borne infectious agents (e.g. hepatitis B, non-A, non-B hepatitis and HIV) to the recipient

With respect to safety, these risks are minimized by extensive donor screening for infectious agents and by the performance during production of a number of validated procedures designed to inactivate viruses (e.g. pH 4, pepsin treatment). However, some risk remains.

All of the above considerations make the possibility of alternative sources of specific antibody increasingly attractive.

POSSIBLE ROLE OF MONOCLONAL ANTIBODIES

Since the development of hybridoma technology by Kohler and Milstein in 1975, monoclonal antibody (Mab)-based products have been widely advocated as an alternative and possibly superior source of antibodies for therapy. There is now a vast repertoire of antigenic specificities to which rodent Mabs are available, many with potential therapeutic applications. These include antibodies to bacterial toxins (e.g. tetanus, endotoxin), to viral antigens (e.g. hepatitis B, CMV, herpes zoster), to lymphocyte subset markers (e.g. CD3 and CD4) and to tumour-specific antigens. The ability to produce hybridoma cell lines of defined specificity to this vast repertoire of antigens permits the extention of the application of serotherapy to a wider range of clinical situations such as cancer and transplantation.

While murine Mabs have already been used therapeutically in these areas, they are not widely used on a routine basis. One of the main obstacles is that repeated administration of rodent immunoglobulin results in the production of human anti-mouse immunoglobulin antibodies (HAMA). These antibodies are both anti-species and specific for the idiotype of the antibody administered and their production effectively reduces the half-life of the murine antibody and may lead to clinical complications.

DEVELOPMENT OF HUMAN MONOCLONAL ANTIBODIES

Since the first reports of murine Mab production, the possibility of manufacturing human Mab reagents has been extensively pursued but with less success. The immortalization of human antibody secreting cells has proved to be more difficult than their rodent counterparts, the main reasons being:

- Unavailability of appropriate lymphoid tissue (e.g. spleen or lymph node)
- Inability to immunize donors with the required antigens
- Lack of appropriate fusion partners
- Poor stability of cell lines

However, there have been numerous reports of human Mabs to a variety of antigens (e.g. CMV, tetanus, Rhesus D antigen, tumour-associated antigens) but this by no means represents a full duplication of the range of specificities to which murine Mabs are available. Despite this, the products of many of the human cell lines which are available may prove to be of great clinical value.

The methodology employed for the production of human Mab-secreting cell lines will be discussed in greater detail later.

ALTERNATIVE STRATEGIES

In the absence of reliable methods for the production of human Mabs, the possibility of producing genetically engineered antibodies, made feasible by recent advances, would seem attractive. The ability to express a genetically engineered antibody of defined specificity may offer significant advantages over conventionally expressed antibody. These include:

- The ability to 'humanize' murine Mabs, thereby improving their immunocompatibility
- The ability to select the appropriate isotype in order that the antibody is able to effect a particular biological function (e.g. complement fixation or ADCC)
- Alteration of affinity or avidity of the engineered antibody
- Use of gene fusion to produce bispecific antibodies
- Higher levels of gene expression
- The possibility of salvaging unstable human Mab secreting cell lines

In addition, in using genetic engineering technology we are not limited to antibodies as they are in nature. Novel proteins that possess the binding properties of an antibody can be created by replacing part or all of the C-region DNA sequence of the immunoglobulin molecule with a sequence from another molecule (e.g. enzyme or toxin) for potential use in immunoassay, drug targeting or tumour imaging.

SAFETY

While the prospect of obtaining antibodies for therapy from alternative sources would seem an attractive solution to many of the problems outlined earlier, it also raises new considerations with respect to the safety of these

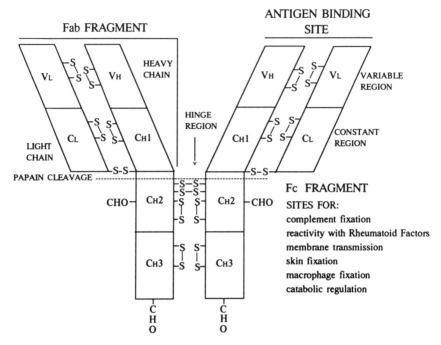

Fig. 8.1. Structure of human immunoglobulin. The four-chain structure of human IgG$_1$, showing disulphide bonds, papain fragments and the location of effector functions. V$_L$ and V$_H$ represent the variable region domains and C$_L$ and C$_{H\ (1-3)}$ represent the constant region domains of the light and heavy chains, respectively. CHO represents carbohydrate

novel therapeutic preparations. The use of Mab-based products for therapy, be they murine, human or 'humanized', produced by the culture of mammalian cells, introduces a new set of hazards including the transfer of viral DNA or viral oncogenes from murine or human myeloma cell lines. Additionally, cytokines (e.g. TNF-1 and IL-1) are produced during the culture of hybridoma and myeloma cells and these contaminants may cause adverse reactions if present in clinical preparations. Therefore, it is necessary that purification protocols be devised and validated to ensure the effective removal or inactivation of such agents. These considerations will be discussed more fully later.

IMMUNOGLOBULIN STRUCTURE AND FUNCTION

GENERAL STRUCTURE

Immunoglobulins are complex glycoproteins with a basic four-chain structure consisting of two heavy and two light chains, the variable domains of

Table 8.2 Human immunoglobulin isotypes

Property*	IgG	IgM	IgA	IgE	IgD
Molecular weight	150000	950000	160000†	190000	175000
Serum concentration (mg/dl)	1250	125	210	0.03	4
% total Ig	75–85	5–10	7–15	0.003	0.3
Half-life (days)	23.0	5.1	5.8	2.5	2.8
Complement fixation	+	+++	–	–	–
Binding to Fc receptors	++	–	–	–	–
Antiviral activity	+++	–	+++	–	–
Antibacterial activity (Gram-negative)	+++	+++††	++††	–	–
Antitoxin activity	+++	–	–	–	–

* +, ++, +++ indicate increasing levels of the denoted activity.
† For monomer.
†† Complement.
††† Lysozyme.

which combine to form the antigen-binding site (Figure 8.1). Various effector functions are mediated by the Fc portion of the molecule, these being isotype-dependent (Table 8.2). The carbohydrate moiety is covalently bound to the heavy chain constant region and has a number of functions including antibody secretion, solubility, protection from degradation and clearance.

ANTIGEN BINDING

Interaction of antibody with antigen occurs at several points, each consisting of 10–12 amino acids, and it is envisaged that the antigen nestles in a groove formed by the variable portion of the heavy and light chains. However, this sequence variability is not uniform and areas of hypervariability known as complementarity-determining regions (CDR) are closely involved in forma-tion of the antigen binding site. These are interspersed by regions of re-stricted variability known as 'framework determinants' (FWR), thought to provide a rigid structure in which the CDR resides. The use of these regions for altering antibody structure will be discussed below.

The ability of an antibody to bind antigen is measured by its affinity. This is an important concept since high- and low-affinity antibodies play differ-ing roles *in vivo*. For example, high-affinity antibodies are superior in neu-tralization of viruses and toxins, in protection from bacterial infection and in the clearance of antigen. Conversely, low-affinity antibodies are implicated in various diseases in which antigen–antibody complexes become deposited in the basement membrane of kidney and lead to impaired renal function.

The term 'avidity' is often used synonymously for 'affinity'. *Affinity* is a thermodynamic expression of the binding energy of antibody for an anti-genic determinant. *Avidity*, however, is more often expressed in terms of the ability of an antibody to effect a biological action such as virus neutraliza-tion, which clearly involves factors other than antibody–antigen binding.

Antibodies can have a wide range of specificities and affinities, this being a function of the hypervariable regions of the molecule. While molecules with similar sequences generally have the same specificity, it is possible for antibodies with differing sequences to bind the same antigen although the affinity is likely to be different. This can arise when an antigen reacts with only a portion of the binding site and can lead to strange cross-reactivities between unrelated antigens. While this is a useful property in defending the body against a range of antigenic challenges, it can lead to problems when immunotherapy is attempted.

IDIOTYPES

The unique sequence of amino acids that makes up the antigen-binding site of an antibody molecule can in its turn become an antigen against which specific antibodies can be formed. These anti-idiotypic antibodies can sometimes block antigen binding. Idiotypic determinants are thought to play an important role in the control of the immune response.

BIOLOGICAL PROPERTIES

Antibodies are the mediators of many important biological functions including neutralization of toxins and viruses, immobilization and agglutination of certain microorganisms and cell lysis in conjunction with complement. Not all isotypes are capable of performing all of these roles and the variations are listed in Table 8.2. Furthermore, certain classes of antibody can be further divided into subclasses in which important functional differences occur. These will now be discussed.

IgG

IgG is the most abundant immunoglobulin in human serum. There are four subclasses of IgG (Table 8.3) and, except for IgG_3, they have the longest half-life *in vivo* of all immunoglobulin isotypes. This makes them the most suitable for passive immunization by transfer of antibodies. IgG (except IgG_2) is the only antibody to pass through the human placenta, via the Fc receptor,

Table 8.3 Human IgG subclasses

Property*	IgG_1	IgG_2	IgG_3	IgG_4
% total IgG	70	20	7	3
Half-life (days)	23	23	7	23
Complement fixation	+++	+	++++	±
Placental passage	++	±	++	++
Fc receptor binding	+++	+	+++	±

±, +, ++, +++ indicate increasing levels of the denoted activity.

thus conferring immunity to the foetus. However, while protecting the foetus from infection it may also be responsible for haemolytic disease of the newborn (HDN) which occurs when maternal antibodies against the Rhesus antigen D on foetal red cells cross the placenta and cause haemolysis.

IgG antibodies are extremely versatile and have a variety of functions such as virus and toxin neutralization, immobilization of bacteria and activation of complement (sub-class dependent, see Table 8.3). They are also good at opsonization of microorganisms and play an important role in ADCC.

IgG molecules can be made to aggregate by a variety of treatments such as heating or alcohol, processes which may be used during purification. Although combination with antigen can still take place, aggregated IgG without antigen can also induce various effects such as activation of complement and other biologically active substances in the body. Thus it is important that no aggregated IgG is present in passively administered antibody.

IgM

IgM is the first immunoglobulin produced in response to an antigenic stimulus and it has a short half-life of 5 days. Its multivalent structure allows IgM to form bridges between distant epitopes and they are thus efficient agglutinating antibodies. Naturally occurring ABO blood-group antibodies are IgM but since IgM does not cross the placenta, they do not harm an incompatible foetus and, indeed, they may offer protection against HDN. IgM antibodies are also very efficient at fixing complement, a single molecule being sufficient to initiate the cascade. However, they are poor at neutralizing toxins or viruses.

IgA

Iga is the major immunoglobulin present in external secretions such as saliva, mucus, sweat, tears, gastric fluid and milk, where it plays an important role in defence against local infections particularly of the respiratory and gastrointestinal tract. The IgA molecule does not contain receptors for complement and therefore cannot induce bacterial lysis. However, in conjunction with lysozyme, IgA does possess bactericidal activity against Gram-negative organisms. Secretory IgA is also efficient at preventing viral entry into cells and is a good agglutinating antibody.

IgE

IgE is present in serum at very low concentrations and has a half-life of only 2.5 days. It reacts like none of the foregoing immunoglobulins and is concerned in both protection of the body against parasites and in mediation of certain hypersensitivity reactions.

IgD

IgD is also found in serum in low amounts but has no known function there. It is, however, present on the surface of many B lymphocytes and serves as a marker of differentiation.

CONVENTIONAL MONOCLONAL ANTIBODIES

RODENT MONOCLONAL ANTIBODIES

As mentioned in the Introduction, monoclonal antibody technology has led to the development of new possibilities for immunotherapy. Mono-clonal antibodies are so called because they are derived from a single antibody-producing cell and the product therefore consists of a pure form of a single antibody, each molecule being identical in structure, specificity and affinity.

Methodology

The basic steps in the production of rodent MAbs are outlined in Figure 8.2. Briefly, animals are hyperimmunized and after a final boost of antigen, the spleen cells (lymphocytes) are extracted and fused with an immortal cell line (myeloma). Under normal culture conditions, lymphocytes will survive for about 2 weeks whereas myeloma cells survive indefinitely, i.e. they are immortal. However, culture conditions are adjusted to ensure that only the product of fusion between a lymphocyte and a myeloma cell, called a 'hybrid', survive. This depends upon the principle that cells can make DNA by two routes: by *de novo* synthesis or by a salvage pathway using pre-formed nucleotides. The drug aminopterin blocks *de novo* synthesis of purines and pyrimidines and when hypoxanthine, aminopterin and thy-midine (HAT) are added to the culture medium, spleen cells containing the enzyme hypoxanthine–guanine phosphoribosyl transferase (HGPRT) can use the salvage pathway, whereas the myeloma cell which is deficient in this enzyme does not survive. Thus only the fusion partnership that combines the HGPRT activity of the lymphocyte with the immortality of the myeloma will grow. This is known as 'HAT selection'. Since the properties of the antibody secreted by the hybrid are derived totally from the lymphocyte, then it is clearly crucial that lymphocytes of the desired specificity have been induced by the immunization regime.

An important feature of the myeloma cell line chosen as fusion partner is that it should not secrete any immunoglobulin; if it did, then its hybrids would continue to express the myeloma heavy and light chains in addition to those of the lymphocyte thus leading to the secretion of mixed antibody

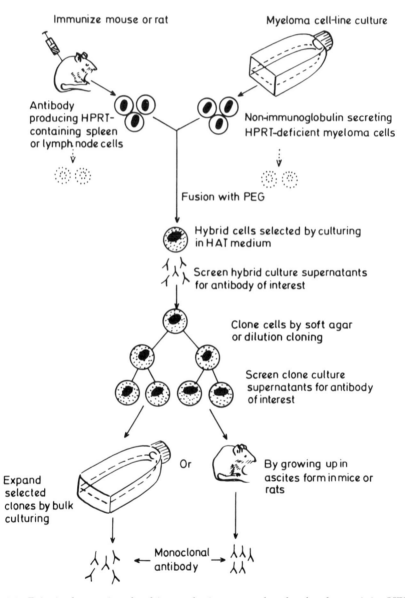

Fig. 8.2. Principal steps involved in producing monoclonals of rodent origin. HPRT = hypoxanthine phosphoribosyl transferase; PEG = polyethyleneglycol. (Reproduced with permission from K. James *et al.* (1984) *Scottish Medical Journal*, **29**, 67–83)

molecules with reduced activity. Nevertheless, this situation can be exploited to create MAbs with dual specificity as will be explained below.

The cells are grown in small wells, one spleen producing sufficient material to seed many hundreds of wells. Culture supernatants are screened

Table 8.4 Examples of clinical uses of murine monoclonal antibodies

Application	Specificity
In vitro bone-marrow depletion	Tumour cells
	T-cell subsets
In vivo tumour imaging	Malignant melanoma
	Mammary carcinoma
	Ovarian carcinoma
Other imaging	Dead heart muscle
Tumour therapy	Malignant melanoma
	Mammary carcinoma
	Ovarian carcinoma
	Lung carcinoma
	Colorectal carcinoma
	T-cell leukaemia
Transplantation rejection	CD3+ T-cells
	CD4+ T-cells
	IL-2 receptor
Growth factor receptors	EGF receptor
	IL-2 receptor
Autoimmune disease	IL-2 receptor
	CD4+ T-cells
Bacterial infection	*Streptococcus mutans*
	Endotoxin
Viral infection	Hepatitis BsAg
	Rhinovirus receptor

against the appropriate antigen by immunoassay and selected hybrids are cloned to ensure true monoclonality. Bulk quantities of MAb can be produced in tissue culture or by growing the cells as an ascitic tumour in mice or rats.

In this way, rodent MAbs have been produced to an immense variety of antigens, some of which are being used or considered for use in humans or have clinical uses *in vitro*. Examples of these applications are listed in Table 8.4.

HUMAN MONOCLONAL ANTIBODIES

The use of the above technology to produce MAbs of human origin has obvious attractions both as an improvement to the plasma-derived preparations available at present and in areas where rodent MAbs may be unsuitable, such as:

- for antigens against which the rodent immune system does not react appropriately, e.g. certain blood-group antigens;
- where there is inefficient triggering of immune effector mechanisms, i.e. incorrect Fc domains; and
- to reduce or eliminate the anti-immunoglobulin reaction.

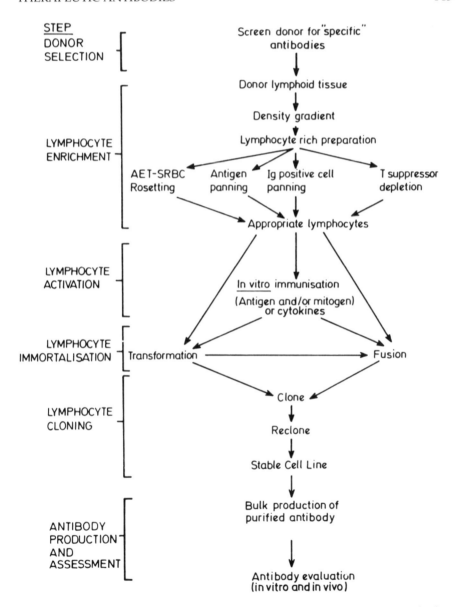

Fig. 8.3. Principal steps in the production of human monoclonal antibodies. AET-SRBC = sheep red-blood cells treated with 3-aminoethylisothiouronium bromide hydrobromide

Unfortunately, a straight transfer of technology has not been possible for the variety of reasons outlined in the Introduction. The principal steps involved in the production of human MAbs are outlined in Figure 8.3 and will be discussed in more detail below.

Immune lymphocytes

Of crucial importance is an adequate supply of immune B lymphocytes in the appropriate state of differentiation and proliferation and, coupled with this, effective methods for immortalizing and cloning them. Although the most convenient source of human lymphocytes is peripheral blood (PBL), many studies have shown these cells to be inferior to those from solid lymphoid tissues. However, a recent innovation has been the treatment of PBL with leucyl-leucine O-methyl (Leu-Leu-O-Me) ester which kills certain suppressor cells while sparing both those with helper functions and the B lymphocytes. The resultant cell mixture can then be stimulated with antigen *in vitro* for several days prior to immortalization or immortalized immediately if derived from a suitable donor.

IMMORTALIZATION OF HUMAN B-CELLS

Fusion

Attempts to repeat the fusion strategy for producing rodent MAbs have been frustrated by the lack of suitable human partners. Since human myeloma cells are generally difficult to grow in culture, alternative lines such as Epstein–Barr virus (EBV)-transformed lymphoblastoid cells (LCL) have been used. However, few of these are non-secretors and they tend to transfer the EBV genome to their hybrids thus causing potential problems in downstream processing of their product. Fusion with murine myelomas is possible and although the resultant hybrids tend to lose preferentially some of the human chromosomes involved in antibody production, the efficiency of fusion is still adequate. As a compromise, several groups have fused murine myelomas with normal human B lymphocytes to produce potential fusion partners with the growth and fusion characteristics of the murine myeloma while retaining sufficient human chromosomes to promote the formation of stable human antibody secreting hybrids derived from immune B-cells.

Virus transformation

Immortalization with EBV is much more efficient than most fusion protocols (around 1 in 10^4 cells compared with 1 in 10^5 to 10^8 for fusion) and has been widely used to produce many valuable cell lines. However, these lines are often difficult to clone, they secrete low amounts of antibody and may cease antibody secretion after several weeks or months in culture. To combat this instability, the antibody-secreting lines can be fused with murine, human or hetero-hybridoma cells. The resultant hybrids tend to grow better in culture, they can be cloned at one cell per well and may even secrete antibody at higher levels.

Table 8.5 Potential therapeutic applications for human MAbs

Infectious disease	Passive therapy
	Enhancement of vaccine response
	Anti-idiotype vaccines
	Identification of immunogenic epitopes
Malignancy	Imaging
	Therapy – alone or as drug–isotope conjugate
	Anti-idiotype vaccines
	Identification of immunogenic epitopes
Autoimmunity	Rhesus incompatibility
	Transplantation rejection
	Immunomodulation
	Anti-idiotype
	Contraception

Thus the general strategy used by many groups to produce human MAbs is to transform immune lymphocytes with EBV and then to fuse them with a suitable partner cell shortly after. This may be preceded by a selection step for antigen-specific cells.

Bulk production

The production of large quantities of human MAbs is generally by *in vitro* methods. Although it is possible to grow these cells as ascitic tumours in mice, the animals have to be immunodeficient (genetically, by irradiation, or both) and the overall yield is low. This coupled with the expensive housing required and the possibility of contamination of the final product by viruses and rodent antibodies tends to make bulk tissue culture the first choice.

POTENTIAL APPLICATIONS OF HUMAN MAbs

The limited experience gained to date using rodent MAbs *in vivo* has suggested wider areas in which human MAbs may have a potential role to play (Table 8.5). Some of these applications will be discussed in greater detail later.

LIMITATIONS

In spite of the progress made in the production of human MAbs, there remain a number of problem areas. Initially, extensive screening may be necessary to identify a suitable donor. The appropriate cells may be present in the circulation for a limited time after boosting and specific suppressor or toxic cells may also be induced. For specificities requiring *in vitro* immunization there may be problems with toxicity or immunosuppressive properties of the antigen.

In general, the methodology available to most laboratories is still relatively inefficient although advances in genetic engineering may circumvent this in future. Likewise, the relatively poor affinity and restricted isotype of human MAbs (commonly IgM) may be improved by similar techniques.

ALTERNATIVE STRATEGIES

The ability to produce Mabs by genetic engineering would obviate many of the problems encountered in using conventional hybridoma technology. Furthermore, the application of genetic engineering methodology to this area may offer additional significant advantages (see Introduction).

EXPRESSION OF IMMUNOGLOBULIN GENES IN BACTERIA AND YEAST

Attempts made to express immunoglobulin (Ig) genes in both bacteria and yeast have largely been unsuccessful. The products obtained from bacterial expression have been found to be insoluble, heterogeneous in size and to exhibit little or no antigen-binding activity. The level of expression was also found to be extremely low (0.5–32 μg/litre). In some instances it is possible to restore some antigen-binding activity by treating the products with denaturing agents which promote disulphide bond interchange; however, this *in vitro* reassembly is extremely inefficient. Additionally, the Ig products obtained were unglycosylated which may have contributed to their insolubility and lack of antigen-binding activity. While there have been a few reports of partial Ig molecules expressed in *E. coli* which were correctly assembled and functional, these remain the exceptions.

Attempts have been made to circumvent some of these problems using yeast to express Ig genes. There would appear to be two major advantages in the use of yeasts:

• The availability of well-developed fermentation technology for scale-up
• Yeasts are capable of asparagine-linked glycosylation though restricted to high mannose carbohydrate

However, although it is possible to express both heavy- and light-chain genes in yeasts with the heavy chain being glycosylated, it was found that the antibody produced exhibited extremely low specific activity with antigen. Therefore, it seems that the addition of high mannose carbohydrate is not sufficient and indeed that high mannose sugars added to multiple sites may disrupt heavy-chain structure.

Additionally, since neither bacteria nor yeast efficiently secrete proteins, the Ig product must be extracted by mechanical disruption of the cell membrane. As a result, these products may be heavily contaminated with either yeast cell-wall components or bacterial endotoxin. Such contaminants could cause adverse clinical reactions (e.g. endotoxic shock). Therefore it becomes necessary to devise suitable downstream processing protocols for the removal of these components to ensure their safety in therapeutic use.

EXPRESSION OF IMMUNOGLOBULIN GENES IN MAMMALIAN LYMPHOID CELLS

The transfection and expression of immunoglobulin genes in mammalian cells would circumvent many of the problems discussed above. The advantages offered by eukaryotic expression include:

- Appropriate assembly and glycosylation of immunoglobulin
- High levels of gene expression and efficient secretory mechanisms
- Safer products

The most common hosts for transfected Ig genes are murine myeloma cell lines (e.g. SP2/0 and P3 X63 Ag8.6.5.3). Even under optimal conditions, transfection frequencies are low (i.e. 1×10^{-4} to 1×10^{-5}) and it is therefore necessary to transfect with vectors expressing biochemically selectable markers in order to facilitate the identification and isolation of stable transfectants. Both electroporation and protoplast fusion have been found to be efficient methods for transfecting DNA into lymphoid cells. The V-region genes are obtained either as cDNA or as genomic clones. An advantage in using genomic clones is that the V-region is obtained as a complete transcription unit with its own promoter and splice junction. A J-region probe can then be used to identify expressed V-region exons since these genes are juxtaposed to a J-region, unlike non-expressed V-genes. This circumvents the need to sequence the gene. Unfortunately, hybridoma cells often contain aberrantly arranged V-region sequences and in these instances further characterization is required. The techniques involved are discussed in greater detail in Chapter 4.

It is possible to design and construct antibody cassette expression vectors so that once a particular V-region is cloned it can easily be placed next to any C-region gene. This facilitates isotype switching to obtain antibodies of the appropriate class or subclass to effect a particular biological function (e.g. complement fixation, ADCC). This represents a major advantage over somatic mutation as a method of isolating class-switch variants, since this work is extremely labour intensive and limited in that it is only possible to switch to isotypes which lie downstream of the original H-chain.

EXPRESSION OF IMMUNOGLOBULIN GENES IN INSECT CELLS

A more recent development is the use of insect cells to express genes coding both for Ig and other proteins. The DNA is inserted into a baculovirus which infects insect cells and the protein is synthesized along with the viral ones.

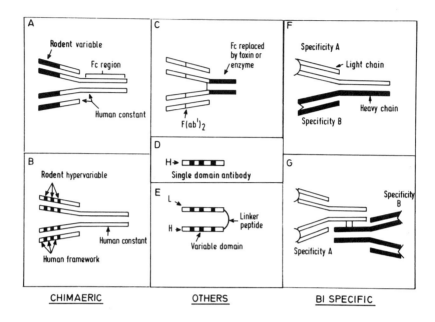

Fig. 8.4. Second-generation monoclonal antibody constructs. These have been produced using genetic-engineering, cell-fusion and chemical techniques. The genetically engineered products include 'humanized' chimaeric (A) and mosaic (B) antibodies, single-determinant (D) and single-chain (E) antibodies. Monovalent antibodies can also be produced by cell fusion between antibody A with the desired activity and an irrelevant specificity B (F). Hybrid molecules have been produced where the Fc portion of the molecule has been replaced by a toxin or enzyme (C). Bispecific antibodies capable of reacting simultaneously with two different antigens (A and B) can be produced by cell fusion (F) or by chemical linkage (G). (Reproduced with permission from K. James (1990) *Seminars in Cancer Biology*, **1**, 243–253)

CHIMAERIC ANTIBODIES

This technology also makes it possible to clone the V-region from a murine antibody and to express this gene with a human C-region of the appropriate isotype to produce a chimaeric antibody (Figure 8.4A). This 'humanization' of murine antibodies is advantageous in that it improves on the immuno-compatibility of the original Mab and permits the production of chimaeric antibodies to the vast repertoire of rodent Mabs which have not been duplicated in the human system. In addition, the human form of the Fc region should improve mediation of antibody effector functions. This same technology can also be used to salvage unstable human Mab secreting cell lines and to effect class switching of human antibodies since it is possible to express complete human Ig molecules in rodent lymphoid cells.

MOSAIC V-REGIONS

Instead of using the entire cDNA V-region or genomic exon it is possible to create mosaic V-regions with the FWR from one source and the CDR from another by sequencing the V-region gene segment, synthesizing the CDR and inserting these sequences into the FWR (Figure 8.4B). Both murine and human, H and L-chain, mosaic V-gene cassettes have been generated. The application of this technique in the humanization of rodent Mabs may be beneficial in producing antibodies for therapy since it reduces the amount of foreign protein sequences introduced and further decreases the immuno-genicity of the product.

SINGLE DETERMINANT ANTIBODIES

There have been reports of the production of single determinant monoclonal antibody molecules consisting of the V_H region only and expressed in bacteria (Figure 8.4D). It has been suggested that these single determinant mono-clonals are 'smaller but smarter'; however it is likely that their usefulness in therapy will be limited since they are monovalent and lack the Fc region necessary to trigger various effector functions (e.g. phagocytosis, ADCC or complement fixation). On the other hand, these features may be advant-ageous in some instances where their inability to trigger effector functions results in antigen blockade (e.g. autoimmunity). Additionally, their mono-valency may prevent antigen capping and re-expression since these mole-cules are unable to cross-link. It is also possible to link these V_H molecules to a single determinant V_L molecule via a linker peptide (Figure 8.4E).

An alternative strategy for the generation of monovalent antibodies is the fusion of a hybrid-cell secreting antibody of the required specificity to a cell line secreting an irrelevant immunoglobulin. The random assembly of Ig chains results in a proportion of the antibody molecules being monovalent for antigen binding. Monovalent antibodies generated by this method have intact Fc pieces. These antibody molecules may be of use in improving complement-mediated cell lysis where conventional bivalent antibodies in-duce modulation of cell-surface antigens rendering them resistant to lysis.

BISPECIFIC ANTIBODIES

The methodology used to generate monovalent antibodies by cell fusion can also be utilized to produce bispecific antibodies by the fusion of two cell lines secreting antibodies of different specificities (Figure 8.4G). This results in a proportion of the antibodies having dual specificity. Bispecific anti-bodies have potential therapeutic applications in drug or toxin targeting where one specificity is directed against the drug or toxin. These antibodies offer advantages over covalently attached antibody–toxin/drug conjugates since it is then possible to administer the two active agents separately thus avoiding aggregate formation. Additionally, bispecific antibody could be used to re-target effector cells *in vivo* which would permit the modulation of normal effector mechanisms. For example, bispecific antibodies with one specificity directed against a tumour cell-associated antigen and the other for the appropriate T-cell antigen (e.g. CD3) may have potential use in improving T-cell killing of the tumour cells *in vivo* since it has been shown that monoclonal antibodies specific for T-cell surface antigens are able to reproduce the signals for activation.

NOVEL ANTIBODY MOLECULES

As stated in the Introduction, one of the possible advantages of genetically engineering antibody molecules is that we are not, as in nature, limited to immunoglobulins. It is now possible to design novel proteins that possess the binding specificity of antibody molecules and sequences derived from another molecule such as an enzyme or toxin (Figure 8.4C). Such entities would have great potential use in immunotherapy for targeting biologically active agents and in tumour imaging. One example of an antibody-targeted pharmacological agent is the expression of the V_H region of an anti-fibrin antibody joined to a mouse G2b constant region that had most of the C-region exons replaced by the sequence encoding the catalytic beta-chain of tissue plasminogen activator (t-PA). This engineered heavy chain was secreted in conjunction with the parent light chain. However, the fusion protein obtained exhibited only 70% of the peptidolytic activity of the native t-PA. In order to produce fully active fusion proteins it may be necessary for the joined molecule to be able to fold independently to reconstitute active domains.

LIMITATIONS

The options made available to us by advances in genetic engineering seem to offer advantages over conventional hybridoma technology since it allows the choice of the class or subclass of the antibody expressed. However, there remain several limitations of this technology which have not been fully resolved.

Levels of product expression

A persistent problem has been the expression level of transfected immuno-globulin genes. While heavy-chain gene expression frequently approaches the levels seen in hybridoma cells, the efficient expression of light-chain genes is more difficult to achieve. The reasons for this disparity in levels of expression remain unclear. Gene amplification has been used to raise the level of immunoglobulin gene expression. However, even after amplification, the level of light chain is generally lower. Further, the level of antibody secreted by transfectants would not, as yet, appear to offer an advantage over hybridoma cells.

Stability of transfected cell lines

One of the major problems in the use of conventional hybridoma technology for the generation of human monoclonal antibody-secreting cell lines has been the low frequency of stable hybrids, although there are ever-increasing numbers of hybrids and heterohybrids which have proved stable in long-term tissue culture. With respect to transfected cell lines, there is little published data to indicate their long-term stability in culture. Until this type of information is available, it is difficult to predict their potential in the manufacture of therapeutic products.

THERAPEUTIC APPLICATIONS

Monoclonal antibodies (Mabs), whatever their source, have enormous potential as immunotherapeutic agents. However, before the translation of any reagent from laboratory into therapeutic use can take place certain requirements must be met. These include:

- Appropriate *in vitro* functional evaluation of the candidate antibodies using appropriate assays of biological efficacy (e.g. virus neutralization, bacterial phagocytosis or target lysis by ADCC). This permits the formulation of a therapeutic preparation suitable for its intended use
- Full characterization of cell lines in terms of growth requirements and microbiological contaminants (viruses, mycoplasma)
- The design of cell-culture systems suitable for pharmaceutical grade manufacture
- Appropriate downstream processing of the product to ensure the removal or inactivation of possible contaminants (e.g. viruses, cytokines and culture supplement components), together with validation of these processes
- Full evaluation of the efficacy and safety of the antibody *in vivo* in both animal models and in clinical trial (e.g. red-cell clearance studies using anti-D intended for use in Rhesus prophylaxis)

While the advent of Mabs offers opportunities for improved and novel immunotherapy, to a large extent their potential is, as yet, unrealized, since few Mab-based preparations are used routinely. The most widely used Mab preparation is the murine antibody OKT-3 which is directed against the

T-cell antigen CD3. This antibody has been used effectively to treat acute allograft reaction following renal and bone-marrow transplantation. However, repeated administration provokes the production of HAMA although this is generally less clinically important than the adverse reaction frequently observed following treatment with polyclonal anti-lymphocyte preparations. The production of such antibodies to OKT-3 reduces the effectiveness of the therapy by preventing binding. More recently, Phase 1 clinical trials have commenced using a humanized antibody with specificity similar to OKT-3 (CAMPATH-1) which may circumvent some of the problems encountered in the use of murine antibodies.

Currently, there are no human Mab-based products in routine use in immunotherapy. One area most likely to benefit by the availability of a human Mab preparation is the prevention of Rhesus HDN by the passive administration of anti-D. A variety of human anti-D Mabs of different immunoglobulin class and subclass are now available with a wide range of biological functions and a number of these antibodies are currently being assessed for their potential usefulness in therapy. Other areas which would benefit from a human Mab-based reagent are those for which there is no specific conventional polyclonal therapy. One such example is an antibody to Gram-negative bacterial endotoxin for the treatment of endotoxic shock and septicaemia.

REGULATION OF THERAPEUTIC PRODUCTS

The recent increase in use of the products of cultured cells for human therapy has stimulated the Office of Biologics Research and Review (OBRR) to compile a list of problems, side-effects, toxicities, etc. of which investigators and clinicians should be aware. In addition, they have distributed a document called *Points to Consider in the Manufacture of Monoclonal Antibody Products for Human Use (1983)*, revised in 1987, which serves as a baseline guide for manufacturers and Regulatory authorities. It contains detailed guidance on the information that the Regulatory authority will require about the development and characterization of the Mab-producing cell line in addition to the purification and characterization of its product.

CELL-LINE CHARACTERIZATION AND PRODUCTION OF MAb

Some of the details required about a cell line are as follows:

- Source, name and characterization of parent cell and any immunoglobulin secreted
- Origin of immune cell
- Identification and characterization of immunogen

- Immunization scheme
- Screening procedures
- Cell-cloning procedures
- Seed-lot system for setting up primary cell seed and working cell bank

Establishment of seed cultures is particularly important and the cells should be well characterized with respect to identity, stability and known microbiological contaminants.

On the production side, a full description of tissue-culture facilities and purification procedures is required:

- Tissue-culture protocol and controls for culture media
- Steps taken to control viral, bacterial and mycoplasma contamination
- Acceptance criteria for cells or supernatants before further production takes place
- Purification procedures
- Preparation, filling and storage of intermediate and final product

Hybridoma stability is particularly important especially as production runs may last over many generations of cells. Any deviation in the antibody secreted is monitored by extending the test culture period beyond that for production and comparing the final antibody with the original.

Purification procedures should ensure that the final product is homogeneous, free from denatured or aggregated antibody, uncontaminated by chemicals leached during purification and that it retains the original antigen-binding properties. Human MAbs are often IgM, an isotype prone to form aggregates during storage, and special formulations may be required to combat this.

QUALITY CONTROL

A standard preparation of MAb must be established against which ensuing lots can be compared for potency and identification. Mutations of secreted antibody can occur and can be tested for using biochemical or biophysical characterization.

Of major concern is the potential presence of viruses or viral nucleic acid in the final product. Murine cells may harbour a vast array of viruses, tests for which must be undertaken by qualified laboratories. Special considerations apply to MAbs of human origin and the master cell bank must be tested for the following viruses:

- Epstein–Barr virus: infectious virus, viral nuclear antigen (EBNA) or DNA hybridization if EBNA negative

• Cytomegalovirus: tissue-culture assay
• Hepatitis B virus: surface antigen (HBsAg) assay
• Retroviruses: reverse transcriptase, electron microscopy, co-cultivation or DNA hybridization for integrated provirus.
• Other viruses: tissue culture safety test on a panel of cell types.

It is recognized that clinically useful MAb-producing cells may harbour viruses and it is therefore recommended that during purification either specific steps are taken to remove both viruses and nucleic acid or the processing is validated as being able to inactivate any viruses. This latter option ensures that unknown or undetectable infectious organisms are accounted for. In addition, following the discovery of clinically important human retroviruses, particularly HIV, lymphocyte donors must be carefully screened especially since an individual can be infected by HIV and remain both asymptomatic and seronegative for some time after infection.

Recent studies have detected the presence in culture supernatants of clinically significant amounts of cytokines such as IL-1, IL-2 and TNF. Thus final product testing must include quantification of these substances as well as of potential contaminants such as antibiotics, chromatography reagents and preservatives. All this is in addition to the standard tests for identity, potency, stability, purity, general safety and pyrogenicity. In cases of life-threatening disease, less-extensive testing may be permitted, although certain viruses must be excluded.

A further set of guidelines covers MAbs coupled with other agents, drugs or radionuclides with the general aim being that the product is safe and efficacious in use.

CONCLUSION

We have attempted here an introduction to the present state of antibodies as therapeutic agents. We have mentioned the problems with currently available polyclonal products and the role that monoclonal antibodies are playing now and might play in future. The successful treatment of patients with certain murine antibodies, particularly in overcoming rejection of transplanted organs, is already providing useful clinical experience in handling these agents. As our understanding of the relationships between protein structure and function improve, so it should become possible to produce on a routine basis 'tailor-made' antibodies or antibody-like molecules. Even within the current state of the technology, the potential uses for both rodent and, in particular, human antibodies remain enormous although this potential has yet to be fully realized. It is to be hoped that research in this area will continue to be funded in order that treatment for so many life-threatening diseases may be advanced.

ACKNOWLEDGEMENT

The authors would like to thank Dr Keith James for his continuing encouragement and support.

FURTHER READING

Boyd, J.E. and James, K. (1988) Development of monoclonal antibodies. In: *Immunological Diagnosis of Sexually Transmitted Diseases* (Eds) H. Young and A. McMillan). Marcel Dekker, New York and Basel.
Byer, V.S. and Baldwin, R.W. (1988) Therapeutic strategies with monoclonal antibodies and immunoconjugates. *Immunology*, **65**, 329–335.
Masuho, Y. (1988) Human monoclonal antibodies: prospects for use as passive immunotherapy. *Serodiagnosis and Immunotherapy in Infectious Disease*, **2**, 319–340.
Morrison, S.L. and Oi, V.T. (1989) Genetically engineered antibody molecules. *Advances in Immunology*, **44**, 65–92.
Steward, M.W. (1984) *Antibodies: Their Structure and Function*. Chapman and Hall, London and New York.

9 Haemoglobin and Albumin

S.L. MacDONALD and SARAH M. MIDDLETON

HAEMOGLOBIN

The need for a red-cell substitute has long been recognized and efforts to develop such a product have intensified over the last ten years largely due to the increased risk of viral disease transmission (HIV, hepatitis) associated with transfusion of human donor blood. These risks may now include elevated infection and cancer recurrence rates secondary to immune-function alterations. In many Third World countries, the handling of donor blood presents problems which could be resolved by the development of a stable oxygen-carrying plasma expander.

Haemoglobin in solution has many characteristics of an ideal plasma expander: oxygen carriage and release, colloid oncotic pressure, absence of blood-group specific antigens (obviating the need for compatibility testing) and a potential shelf-life exceeding that of intact donor erythrocytes. Traditional plasma expanders such as isotonic saline and Ringer's lactate, together with the iso-oncotic colloid suspensions (dextran, 5% albumin, hetastarch), deliver no oxygen beyond that carried in simple solution.

It is envisaged that a haemoglobin-based plasma expander could reduce the homologous whole-blood requirement in a large proportion (approximately 60%) of surgical patients and in cases of acute blood loss. This would not include patients with a diminished blood flow to the heart or with a pre-existing severe anaemia. Such a product may also be of value in cardiopulmonary bypass procedures, balloon angioplasty (where the reduced viscosity would be an advantage) and in cancer surgery where there is now growing evidence that homologous blood transfusion can adversely affect the immune system.

STRUCTURE AND FUNCTION

Haemoglobin is a tetrameric protein with an overall molecular weight of 67 kDa and comprising two α and two β chains: the α and β-subunits contain 141 and 146 amino acid residues, respectively. Each subunit contains a haem group arranged in such a way that the four haem groups are equidistant

Plasma and Recombinant Blood Products in Medical Therapy
Edited by C.V. Prowse.   Published 1992 by John Wiley & Sons Ltd

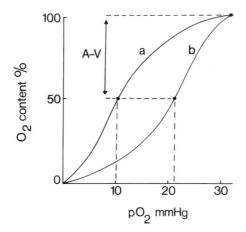

Fig. 9.1. Oxygen saturation curves. The increased oxygen affinity of SFH (a) compared the normal whole blood (b) will result in the delivery of less oxygen to the tissues at any given pO_2 and a reduced venous oxygen pressure when the arteriovenous (A-V) oxygen difference remains constant

from one another. At the centre of each haem is an iron atom to which oxygen, or another ligand, binds reversibly. Haem is linked to the protein part of the subunit by a covalent bond between the iron atom and a histidine residue, known as the 'proximal histidine'.

Haemoglobin tetramer in free solution will tend to dissociate into $\alpha\beta$ dimers which are sufficiently small to be rapidly lost from the circulation into urine, and may have adverse effects on the kidney.

The amount of oxygen which a given amount of haemoglobin takes up is a function of the partial pressure of oxygen (pO_2) with which it is in contact. Each haem group has one binding site and so the tetramer can bind up to four molecules of oxygen. When some of these binding sites combine with oxygen, the protein subunits rearrange themselves in such a way that the overall affinity of the remaining haem groups for oxygen is increased. This cooperation between haem groups in binding oxygen is an example of an allosteric effect and gives rise to the characteristic sigmoid shape of the oxygen dissociation curve (Figure 9.1).

To dissociate half the bound oxygen from arterial blood, the pO_2 need only be reduced to 24 mmHg (at 37°C and pH 7.4) and this allows the tissues to function at relatively high oxygen tension without limiting too severely the amount of oxygen which is delivered.

FACTORS WHICH AFFECT OXYGEN AFFINITY

When fully saturated, 1 g of haemoglobin can transport 1.34 ml of oxygen. However, the position of the oxygen dissociation curve and, hence, the

50% saturation point (p50) depends upon several factors. Early investigators found that a fall in pH will shift the curve to the right and so lower oxygen affinity. This is known as the 'Bohr effect'. The lower pCO_2 found in the lungs will therefore favour the binding of oxygen where the pO_2 is highest. Active tissue has a high pCO_2, low pH, raised temperature and all of these changes will bring about greater release of oxygen for respiratory processes.

The allosteric effector molecule 2,3 diphosphoglycerate (2,3-DPG) is found within the intact human erythrocyte. Chemical and X-ray diffraction studies have shown that 2,3-DPG binds electrostatically to β-subunits through lysine-82, histidine-143 and the N-terminal groups. Only in the deoxygenated haemoglobin configuration are these groups arranged so as to allow binding of 2,3-DPG. During oxygenation, the cleft between β-chains closes and 2,3-DPG is expelled. This molecule is therefore an effective inhibitor of oxygen binding and will cause haemoglobin to unload oxygen. Reduced levels of 2,3-DPG cause an overall increase in oxygen affinity and this has the most profound implications for the ability of haemoglobin in free solution effectively to unload oxygen in the tissues.

INFUSION OF UNMODIFIED HAEMOGLOBIN SOLUTION

Infusion of 'stroma-free' haemoglobin solution in the earlier part of this century was associated with marked vasoconstriction and a transient reduction in renal function. These adverse reactions have now been attributed to the presence of contaminating stromal elements and haemoglobin solutions prepared today, by various methods, tend to retain <1% of the original stromal lipid.

Total exchange transfusion of stroma-free haemoglobin (SFH) solution into adult baboons during the mid-1970s showed that all animals could survive to zero haematocrit. In contrast, control animals exchanged with Dextran-70 died at a haematocrit of 5%. Moreover, there were significant differences in the way the two groups of animals responded during the exchange. The Dextran-treated animals responded to isovolaemic anaemia by an elevated cardiac output and increased oxygen extraction. This led to a decrease in the tension at which oxygen is unloaded in the tissues (pVO_2). However, the haemoglobin-treated baboons showed no increase in cardiac output and succeeded in maintaining near normal oxygen consumption solely by increased oxygen extraction resulting in a reduced pVO_2. Figure 9.1 demonstrates that if the arterio-venous oxygen difference (A–V) remains unchanged, the increased oxygen affinity found in haemoglobin solutions (the left shifted curve) must inevitably lead to reduced pVO_2 levels. As this is considered to reflect reduced tissue oxygen reserves, this finding was viewed with some alarm and prompted efforts to normalize the oxygen affinity of infused haemoglobin solutions.

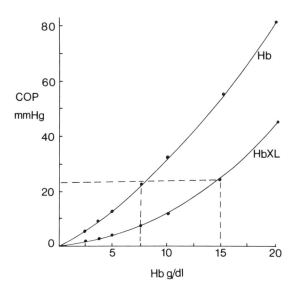

Fig. 9.2. Colloid oncotic pressure of stroma-free haemoglobin (Hb) and pyridoxa-lated polymerized haemoglobin (HbXL). Polymerization allows the haemoglobin concentration to be increased from 7.5 to 15 g/dl while maintaining the colloid oncotic pressure (COP) at the physiological level of 20–25 mmHg

The addition of 2,3-DPG to haemoglobin in solution produced disappointing results due to the rapid loss of 2,3-DPG from the circulation. However, the covalent linkage of pyridoxal phosphate (PLP) into the 2,3-DPG binding site located in the cleft between β-chains produced a permanent reduction in oxygen affinity and was first described by Benesch in the mid-1970s. Infusion of pyridoxalated haemoglobin into the baboon exchange transfusion model resulted in significantly raised whole blood p50 levels compared to those given by unmodified haemoglobin solution. However, the tissue pO_2 still remained below that found in normal control animals.

The need to maintain a normal colloid oncotic pressure (COP) had required that the haemoglobin concentration not exceed 7 g/dl in the infused solutions. Attempts to normalize the pVO_2 therefore concentrated on increasing the haemoglobin concentration whilst maintaining a normal COP and this was achieved by polymerization of the haemoglobin tetramers. Figure 9.2 shows the relationship between COP and haemoglobin concentration in both pyridoxalated haemoglobin (Hb) and pyridoxalated, polymerized haemoglobin (HbXL). Normal plasma COP is between 20–25 mmHg and polymerization allows this value to be maintained whilst also increasing the haemoglobin concentration from 7.5 to 15 g/dl. Cross-linking also prevents dissociation of haemoglobin tetramers into dimers and the resultant excretion of haemoglobin into urine.

APPROACHES TO MODIFICATION AND POLYMERIZATION

Pyridoxal phosphate (PLP)

The finding that pyridoxal derivatives could be used to effect permanent changes in the oxygen affinity of haemoglobin solved one of the major problems in the development of haemoglobin-based red-cell substitutes as described above. Pyridoxalation is confined to the N-terminal amino groups of β-chains if the haemoglobin is in the deoxy conformation and this results in a reduced oxygen affinity. Modification of oxygenated, or liganded, haemoglobin results in modification of the α-chain N-terminal amino groups and a raised oxygen affinity.

Glyoxylic acid

The covalent linkage of glyoxylic acid to haemoglobin in the oxygenated conformation will effect a reduction in oxygen affinity. However, this apparent advantage is made less useful by the finding that prior modification with glyoxylic acid reduces the effectiveness of subsequent polymerization with some crosslinking agents. This problem is resolved by glyoxylating deoxygenated haemoglobin but this removes the major advantage offered by this agent over PLP – namely, removal of the need to thoroughly deoxygenate before the reaction can proceed.

2-Nor-2-formylpyridoxal 5'-phosphate (NF-PLP)

NF-PLP is a derivative of PLP which blocks dissociation of tetrameric haemoglobin into the dimer form by covalent coupling between β-chains in the deoxy state whilst simultaneously reducing oxygen affinity. The circulatory half-life is therefore prolonged and renal excretion minimized. This approach to modification has received much attention but the compound is both time-consuming and difficult to synthesize which may explain why it has not become available from commercial sources in the 15 years since it was first studied.

Bis-pyridoxal tetraphosphate (bis-PLP)

Bis-PLP represents one of a series of recently synthesized intramolecular crosslinking agents. The modified product resembles that produced by NF-PLP modification but the chemical synthesis does not present so many complications and may therefore become commercially available.

3,5-Dibromosalicyl-bis-fumarate (DBBF)

The diaspirin reagent DBBF may be used to selectively crosslink α-chains in deoxygenated haemoglobin and bring about a simultaneous reduction in oxygen affinity to physiological levels. As with bis-PLP, this approach is currently receiving a good deal of attention.

Conformation specific stabilizer and crosslinker (CSSC)

These CSSC agents are polyaldehyde derivatives of ring-opened sugars. It is likely that all sugar compounds with between two and seven sugar residues (including particularly raffinose) are potential stabilizing and polymerizing agents and their specific application in the field of haemoglobin-based blood substitutes is now under patent (Hemosol, Canada). It is probable that a haemoglobin product produced using this method will involve use of ring-opening oxidation of raffinose to cross-link within monomeric haemoglobin. This product may then be further polymerized, using a lower cross-linker:haemoglobin ratio, to increase the overall molecular weight.

Coupling pyridoxalated haemoglobin to high-molecular-weight compounds

In order to prolong circulatory half-life, various attempts have been made to complex modified haemoglobin to compounds such as polyethyleneglycol, dextran and insulin. However, such complexes have tended to have a final oxygen affinity too high to be physiologically useful. One very promising recent approach has been to couple pyridoxalated haemoglobin with the activated ester of polyoxyethylene yielding a final conjugate with a mean molecular weight of 90 kDa. The final product is sufficiently robust to withstand pasteurization and lyophilization without the formation of excess methaemoglobin.

Polymerizing agents

Glutaraldehyde

To date, glutaraldehyde has been used by several groups to promote inter-tetramer crosslinking and to introduce a degree of viral kill in the production process. The crosslinking would seem to involve mainly lysine residues of both globin chains and the resulting product is a heterogeneous mixture containing polymers ranging from two to ten crosslinked tetramers, as well as a sizeable proportion of the final product which remains unpolymerized. This heterogeneity introduces problems with regard to batch-to-batch reproducibility and quality control. It is also necessary to remove the unpolymerized fraction from the final product to prevent renal excretion. There are also other problems now associated with dimeric haemoglobin which will be discussed in relation to toxicity.

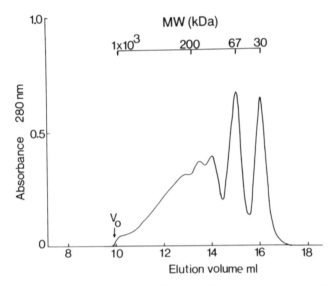

Fig. 9.3. Molecular-weight distribution of glycolaldehyde polymerized haemoglobin solution. The sample has been eluted in 1 M $MgCl_2$ which produces dissociation of the unpolymerized fraction into $\alpha\beta$ dimers. This fraction is removed from the final product to avoid prevent renal excretion. V_O indicates the excluded volume. For the study shown any molecules larger than 1000 kDa would elute at this position

Glycolaldehyde

The bifunctional crosslinking reagent glycolaldehyde represents a class of compounds which offer some promise as crosslinkers of haemoglobin solutions. The reaction involves Amadori rearrangement of Schiff bases and introduces a crosslink predominantly between lysine residues of the β-chains in tetrameric haemoglobin ($\alpha : \beta$ ratio = 30:70). The reaction is extremely reproducible and may be terminated by addition of a reducing reagent. It also has the advantage of allowing polymerization and pyridoxalation to proceed simultaneously, which greatly simplifies production. It also requires that the unpolymerized fraction be removed from the final product. Figure 9.3 shows the typical molecular-weight profile of pyridoxalated haemoglobin polymerized using glycolaldehyde. The peak which elutes at 30 kDa represents the unpolymerized fraction which it is necessary to remove so as to prevent renal excretion and possible nephrotoxicity (discussed below).

Unfortunately, glycolaldehyde does not provide the same degree of viral inactivation as glutaraldehyde in the production process.

Figure 9.4 shows the appearance of NFPLP and glycolaldehyde polymerized human haemoglobin following sodium dodecyl sulphate polyacrylamide gel

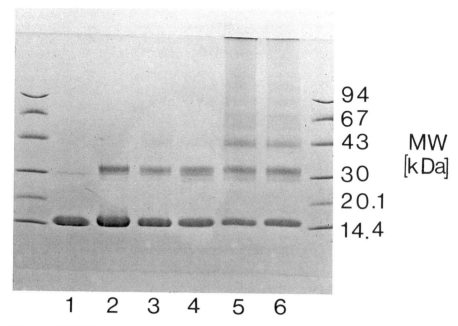

Fig. 9.4. SDS-PAGE electrophoresis (gradient 8–25%) of polymerized haemoglobin solutions. Lanes: (1) represents unpolymerized stroma-free haemoglobin; (2) represents haemoglobin covalently crosslinked between β-chains using NF-PLP; (3) + (4) and (5) + (6) represent haemoglobin lightly and heavily crosslinked, respectively, using the bifunctional reagent glycolaldehyde

electrophoresis (SDS-PAGE). Under these conditions, uncrosslinked globin chains are separated and appear as 15-kDa monomeric subunits.

The general characteristics of pyridoxalated polymerized human haemoglobin solution are shown in Table 9.1.

Table 9.1 Characteristics of polymerized pyridoxalated haemoglobin

Component	Concentration
Haemoglobin	12–15 g/dl
Methaemoglobin	<10%
Molecular weight distribution	68–600 kDa
p50	20–25 mmHg
Binding coefficient	1.30 cc O_2/g Hb
Colloid oncotic pressure	20–25 mmHg
Osmolality	290–310 mOsm/kg
Total phospholipid*	<0.1 mg/dl
Viscosity	2–3 cp (7 g/dl)
Non-haem protein (% of total protein)	<2%

* Total phospholipid assayed by thin-layer and gas–liquid chromatography.

BARRIERS TO CLINICAL TRIALS

Nephrotoxicity was reported in early studies after infusion of haemoglobin solution. This has been attributed to the presence of residual stroma which produced thrombosis of the small renal vasculature. Infusion of stroma-free haemoglobin into dogs was reported to cause no deterioration in renal function.

However, a report by Savitsky *et al.* in 1978 reported the findings of a human clinical safety trial using stroma-free haemoglobin solution which had a chilling effect upon further trials. Eight healthy male volunteers received a 250-ml infusion of haemoglobin solution at a rate of 2–4 ml/min. A transient deterioration in kidney function was noted, evidenced by a decline in creatinine clearance and urine volume. Two albumin control subjects showed no such changes.

Savitsky *et al.* proposed three possible explanations. The first was that residual stroma might be responsible but, in view of the fact that this represented only 1% of the original level and disseminated intravascular coagulation was not seen, this would seem unlikely. The second possibility involved the presence of a vasoactive substance which transiently reduced renal flow. The third explanation was that filtration of haemoglobin dimers (molecular weight 30 kDa) into the kidney produced the changes in renal function. Once the haemoglobinuria had disappeared, renal function returned to normal. This last possibility has prompted most workers to remove all unpolymerized haemoglobin from the final preparation and, indeed, it is reported that nephrotoxicity is much reduced in such preparations.

Vasoactivity

There are many reports of purified haemoglobin solutions producing vasoconstriction in both isolated organ perfusion experiments and intact animal models. However, haemoglobin solutions are produced using a variety of methods and may not all represent the same degree of purity. Certain red cell-derived contaminants, such as the adenine nucleotides, are potent vasoactive agents and, unless total removal is ensured, it is impossible to ascribe vasoactive side-effects directly to the haemoglobin molecule itself. However, it is known that haemoglobin specifically inhibits a factor normally produced by endothelial cells, endothelium-derived relaxing fator (EDRF). It is suggested that this may be responsible for the acute vasospasm commonly associated with sub-arachnoid haemorrhage. Polymerized haemoglobin is not as potent in its effect and reinforces the importance of removing unpolymerized haemoglobin from the final product in order to avoid complications arising should free haemoglobin cross the blood–brain barrier.

Reticuloendothelial system

The main route of excretion is probably the reticuloendothelial system (RES) and a major area of concern is immunosuppression following infusion of polymerized haemoglobin. Sepsis is potentially a very serious complication in patients and it is vital that the haemoglobin does not in any way compromise the host defence mechanism.

There are reports that haemoglobin can promote experimental peritonitis in rats. Granulocyte phagocytosis and bacterial killing are diminished although this was noted only when haemoglobin was injected directly into the peritoneal cavity. No such diminution in defence mechanisms was noted when injection was via intravenous or intramuscular routes.

Whether polymerized haemoglobin can reduce immunocompetence is unclear at present. It is known that the presence of haemoglobin does enhance the toxicity of (Gram-negative) bacteria and may produce depletion of plasma fibronectin levels.

Coagulation

There were early reports that 'stroma-free' haemoglobin solution produced alterations in the coagulation system. However, studies with pure haemoglobin (free of stromal lipid, endotoxin and very high-molecular-weight polymers) have revealed no alteration in coagulation parameters.

There still remain significant barriers to human clinical trials, the most important of which centre on nephrotoxicity and immunosuppression. Much effort is presently being directed towards resolving these issues.

ALTERNATIVE APPROACHES

Bovine haemoglobin

The use of bovine haemoglobin, rather than human haemoglobin, as a source material is an approach receiving serious attention in the USA and has resulted in a product now in the initial stages of human clinical trials (Biopure Corporation, Boston). The raw material is available in large quantity from either the slaughterhouse or a dedicated herd of cows. Biopure estimate that the supply of outdated donor blood in the USA would be insufficient to meet the total demand for a blood substitute product.

Bovine haemoglobin requires no modification to achieve a p50 close to the human norm because oxygen binding and release is controlled by chloride ion concentration rather than 2,3-DPG. The final product is polymerized with glutaraldehyde with a final p50 of 21–24 mmHg and a COP of 20 mmHg at a haemoglobin concentration of 14 g/dl.

Animal studies revealed transient renal toxicity, as evidenced by changes in serum creatinine, as well as accompanying changes in renal histopathology at very high doses. Low-dose levels are reported to produce no such effects. The product has also been reported to produce a 'mild immune response' in primates, presumably on first infusion. There are no reports of re-infusion of bovine haemoglobin into primates although recent studies suggest that when previously immunized rats were given a low-dose re-infusion of bovine (or human) haemoglobin, a severe anaphylactic response was obtained. Specific anti-haemoglobin antibody formation was found.

At present, therefore, there are serious doubts about the possible immunogenicity of haemoglobin derived from non-human sources on repeat infusion.

Liposome-encapsulated haemoglobin (LEH)

The initial concept of encapsulating haemoglobin within an 'artificial red cell' was proposed in the late 1950s since when LEH has evolved into a product proven to carry and deliver oxygen, survive for a reasonable time in the circulation and is amenable to large-scale production. The formation of the liposome has evolved from egg-lecithin and cholesterol mixtures to synthetic distearoylphosphatidylcholine-based blends.

Circulatory persistence and clearance

The size of the liposomes largely determines their physiological fate. Various light-scattering techniques are now used to determine average sizes and these range from 0.3 μm to 0.5 μm. Recent LEH preparations have half-lives of 5–20 h in mice and reports suggest that LEH is predominantly cleared from the circulation by RES uptake in the liver and spleen. This does raise the possibility that massive LEH infusion could saturate the RES and seriously compromise the immune system.

One approach towards improvement of LEH is to alter the liposome surface so as to increase biocompatibility. This has involved the inclusion of carbohydrate moieties resembling those expressed on the red-cell surface and has resulted in increased circulation times. Such LEH preparations may have a reduced impact on the RES system.

Despite the vast amount of work which remains to be done on LEH development, it remains a very promising approach to the eventual successful development of an oxygen-carrying fluid.

Perfluorocarbon emulsions (PFCs)

Perfluorocarbon emulsions are inert, fluorinated hydrocarbons. Traditionally, they have been used as industrial refrigeration fluids and aerosol propellants. However, their capacity to carry both oxygen and carbon dioxide – coupled with a demonstration in the 1970s by Leland Clark of their ability completely to replace blood in rats – led to the production in 1978 of an emulsion called Fluosol-DA 20% (Green Cross Corporation, Japan). This is a 20% blend of perfluorodecalin and perfluorotripropylamine emulsified in a saline solution. This has been tested in a number of clinical situations and, although initial reports on 186 patients suggested no problems, subsequent reports have noted adverse reactions including transient hypotension, leukopenia and pulmonary insufficiency.

There are two major difficulties in the use of PFCs. Firstly, some adverse reactions may reflect complement activation and RES blockade. Secondly, the oxygen dissociation curve of these compounds is linear which means that very high levels of inspired oxygen are necessary for physiological levels of oxygen carriage. In addition to this being an inconvenience, the inspiration of pure oxygen for extended periods of time is believed to be harmful to the lungs.

Researchers are now developing a second generation of PFC emulsions which may overcome these serious problems. These include encapsulating fluorocarbons and thereby avoiding the need for the emulsifying agents which are believed to have been responsible for complement activation.

PFC emulsions do offer great promise for the future but, to date, their usefulness has been limited by lack of efficacy and toxicity.

SOURCES OF HAEMOGLOBIN

Outdated human red cells

The National Statistics for 1988/1989 report that some 66 000 units of red cell concentrate were outdated each year in the Scottish National Blood Transfusion Service (SNBTS). On present production process yield figures for haemoglobin solution (65%), it is estimated that the SNBTS could be self-sufficient until more than 50% of the total demand (approximately all surgical use) is in the form of haemoglobin solution.

Genetic engineering

It is also appropriate to consider whether recombinant DNA technology could be exploited for the provision of an alternative source of the protein. It can be calculated that to replace the current world supply of human red cells would require the production of in excess of 2000 tonnes of recombinant haemoglobin. At the research level, functionally active haemoglobin tetramer has been produced in genetically engineered *Escherichia coli* and *Saccharomyces cerevisiae* and in transgenic mice. Whilst the development of such recombinant haemoglobin is very exciting, a not insignificant challenge lies in progressing from the small-scale expression of limited amounts of recombinant protein, to an economically viable production process.

The problems of achieving economical production of high volume, relatively low cost therapeutic protein using recombinant DNA technology are already being addressed with respect to another plasma expander, human albumin (see below).

CONCLUSION

A prerequisite to any routine clinical use of either haemoglobin-based plasma expanders or PFC emulsions is a better understanding of their effect on normal physiological processes. Both products have progressed to human trials but questions concerning long-term toxicity and immunogenicity remain unanswered. Further studies involving highly purified and standardized preparations are required before further human trials can be conducted. However, there is now clear evidence that an oxygen-carrying plasma expander – as an alternative to donor red cell infusion – is a realizable goal in the not too distant future.

ALBUMIN

STRUCTURE AND FUNCTION

Albumin is the most abundant protein in blood plasma and is the principal protein contributing to the osmolarity of whole blood. It also functions as a major transport protein for endogenous and exogenous compounds. Albumin is synthesized in the liver, and approximately 40% of the exchangeable albumin pool is located in the plasma compartment at a concentration of 40 mg/ml. The remainder is distributed at extravascular sites such as skin, muscle, lungs and other viscera.

In common with serum albumin from other species, human albumin has a very high α-helix content, a high cysteine content and a molecular weight of approximately 66 KDa. It has a relatively low intrinsic viscosity and a strong internal structure held together by 17 disulphide bonds. In its native state it is a highly soluble molecule carrying a strong net negative charge, causing it to migrate rapidly in the appropriate electrophoretic fields. The isoelectric point of the protein is between pH 5.2 and 4.8. Estimates can vary depending on the ligands bound to the protein.

The amino acid sequence for human albumin was first derived by direct protein sequencing and was confirmed, once the gene had been cloned, by deducing the protein sequence from the nucleotide sequence of the cDNA or genomic clones. The molecule contains 585 amino acids in a single chain, and analysis shows an abundance of aspartic and glutamic acid residues;

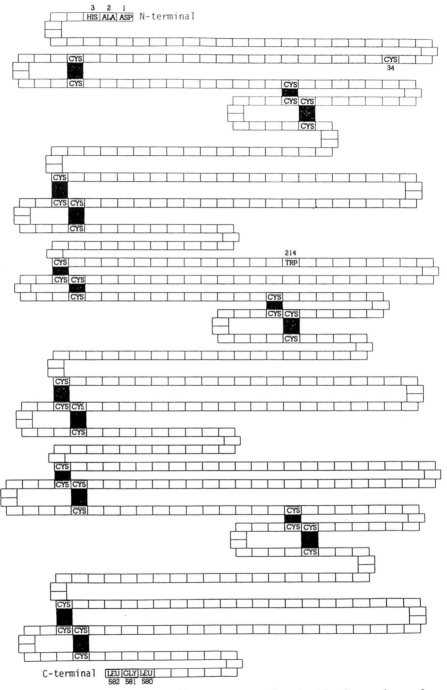

Fig. 9.5. The primary structure of human serum albumin. The figure shows the folding around the disulphide bridges, the free sulphydryl at position 34 and the lone tryptophan at position 214

unusually there is only one tryptophan residue; this is at position 214. There are 34 cysteine residues involved in disulphide bond formation, with one free cysteine residue remaining at position 34 (Figure 9.5). Only haemoglobin has more known structural variants than human albumin; however, unlike haemoglobin, no pathology is observed with albumin variants. Polymorphisms, which are normally single-point mutations, are usually detected through a difference in mobility on electrophoresis. The frequency of variant albumins is often quoted as between 1/3000th and 1/10000th of the population, but this may be an underestimate since relatively specific local surveys have been conducted to date. In the 1970s the secondary and tertiary structure of the protein were deduced by consideration of the amino acid sequence.

It was predicted that the peptide chain is probably folded into nine peptide loops by the disulphide bonds. The content of the α-helices is between 45 and 75%, while the content of the β-sheet is probably below 18%. There is considerable evidence to suggest that the protein is organized into a domain structure – a concept further developed by building three-dimensional models. The models were based on the regular arrangement of cysteine residues, the location of helices and the arrangement of proline residues.

The peptide loops are organized in six half domains (sub-domains) each organized in antiparallel α-helices, forming a hydrophilic outer surface with an inner hydrophobic trough-like structure. The half domains are combined two by two, forming three domains, each containing a narrow hydrophobic channel, which is actually an ideal binding site for the hydrocarbon chain of a fatty acid. However, while this spatial model is particularly appropriate for fatty acid binding, other arrangements of the protein are needed to explain the binding of other entities.

Albumin binds a wide variety of substances ranging from metals, such as copper, nickel and calcium, to fatty acids, amino acids, hormones and an impressive array of drugs. The kinetics of binding of these entities have been studied in an attempt at quantitative and qualitative assessment of binding sites on the protein.

In 1989 human albumin was successfully crystallized, enabling for the first time crystallographic resolution of the three-dimensional structure. The preliminary data obtained using this technique is corroborating the structure predicted from the earlier theoretical models and is providing fresh information with regard to binding sites.

THERAPEUTIC USE

As early as 1837 it was predicted that albumin was needed for transporting metabolites, for maintaining fluidity of the vascular system and for preventing oedema. To the present day, this statement still holds true with respect to therapeutic use. In the clinics, the oncotic role of albumin is still the most widely utilized, albumin solutions being principally indicated in acute and chronic hypovolaemia and obligatory sequestration of the extravascular fluid. The effect of the low intrinsic viscosity of albumin is utilized in priming of pumps for both haemodialysis and cardiac pulmonary bypass. The binding and transport of bilirubin by albumin is to a limited extent applied in the treatment of haemolytic disease of the newborn.

Solutions of human albumin for therapeutic purposes were first developed during the Second World War, to supply a stable resuscitation fluid for use in the battlefield. Today, to satisfy clinical demand, up to 250 tonnes of human albumin are recovered from the fractionation of large pools of plasma. Typically, such human serum albumin (HSA) is supplied as an isotonic sterile solution containing 5, 20 or 25% (w/v) protein. The albumin constitutes $\geq$ 95–96% of the total protein; by contrast, in plasma protein fraction (PPF), a 5% protein solution, albumin may constitute as little as 85% of the total protein. To inactivate blood-borne viruses, albumin solutions are routinely heated at 60°C for 10 h, in the presence of stabilizing ligands.

HUMAN BLOOD AS A SOURCE OF ALBUMIN

The impact of blood-borne viruses has economic, as well as safety implications, on the use of human blood as a source of protein. The implimentation of procedures for viral inactivation reduces yields of the high value Factor VIII protein, necessitating fractionation of over 10 million litres of human plasma, to produce the 1.2 billion units required to meet clinical demand. This is well in excess of the volume of plasma required to satisfy the world's requirement for albumin, the immunoglobulins and Factor IX. Factor VIII, therefore, can be said to drive the plasma fractionation industry.

The effect of the AIDS pandemic has been to accelerate the effort to replace human blood as a source of high risk products. When newly developed recombinant Factor VIII comes onto the market it is likely to unbalance the plasma fractionation equation to the extent that human plasma will become a less economically attractive source of albumin.

The question is, if recombinant DNA technology proves to be an alternative method for supplying Factor VIII, can the same technology be applied to the production of albumin? Without a doubt, *in vitro* production of the two proteins represents vastly different problems.

RECOMBINANT DNA TECHNOLOGY AS A SOURCE OF ALBUMIN

The HSA market is very high volume, at 250 tonnes, compared to Factor VIII, where worldwide clinical demand could be met by the supply of 2–3 kg of the protein. A single minimum dose of albumin is 10–12.5 g; not surprisingly, it has a relatively low selling price, currently (1991) of the order of £2 per gram. Compare this to Factor VIII where the market value of 1 gram of protein is approximately £1.2 million, and a single dose is only 200 μg.

The *in vitro* production of human Factor VIII is currently being developed using mammalian cell culture. Mammalian cells are required to process accurately the large single-chain glycoprotein, but fastidious culture requirements and slow growth make such a system complex and expensive. This system would be totally uneconomical for albumin, where high production volume and low production costs are crucial.

The obvious alternative, for bulk production of proteins, is a microorganism which is relatively easy and cheap to grow. However, on the negative side, some microorganisms may not have the complex biochemistry to accurately carry our post-translational modifications, such as accurate glycosylation or cleavage of protein precursor sequences.

Clearly, in terms of developing an economic production process, it is right to be equally concerned about efficient protein synthesis and efficient protein processing. In view of these harsh economic constraints, it is perhaps not surprising that although the albumin cDNA was one of the first to be cloned, by a group at Genentech in 1981, development of viable production processes have been slow to follow.

THE PROKARYOTES

The physiology and genetics of bacteria are well understood, and indeed bacterial hosts have proved useful for the production of quite small heterologous proteins, such as interferon and human growth hormone. Both *Escherichia coli* and *Bacillus subtilis* have been evaluated as production organisms for human albumin.

Escherichia coli

In common with other Gram-negative bacteria, *E. coli* has a lipopolysaccharide-rich outer membrane, which forms a barrier to exporting cell protein. However, it has been shown that some proteins, such as human growth hormone, can be 'secreted' into the periplasmic space which lies between the inner cytoplasmic membrane and the outer membrane. Attempts have been made to produce human albumin intracellularly, thus taking advantage of potential high productivity. It was found that the protein accumulated inside the cell as insoluble denatured albumin, presumably due to the low redox potential of the intracellular environment. However, it was demonstrated that the protein could be solubilized and renatured successfully using extreme denaturing and reducing conditions, prior to renaturation. Characterization of the renatured albumin showed that the protein had an additional methionine residue at the amino terminal. All mammalian genes have an ATG initiator codon immediately upstream of the N-terminal, which is required to initiate protein translation. *E. coli* lacks the mechanism for cleavage of the methionine, coded for by ATG, from the N-terminal aspartate residue of human albumin. Interestingly enough, further characterization of the Met-albumin implied structural identity with the serum albumin by a number of criteria. The protein appeared to fold correctly around the disulphide bonds and was apparently immunologically identical. The Met-albumin also exhibited normal charge characteristics, with an isoelectic point indistinguishable from serum albumin.

Although recovery of the insoluble protein could be achieved, technically it is not a trivial exercise to denature and renature a protein with such a large number of disulphide bonds, particularly at the large scale. The cost of operating such a process is commercially prohibitive. As a consequence, attempts were made to 'secrete' the protein into the periplasmic space, with the aim of obtaining soluble, partially purified protein. In the event, significant productivity was not achieved – probably due to the large molecular weight and relative complexity of the albumin molecule.

An additional problem to the use of a Gram-negative organism is the presence of the outer lipopolysaccharide-rich membrane. This is normally disrupted, to recover albumin from the cell or periplasm, releasing lipopolysaccharide (endotoxin) which as a potential contaminant places severe demands on the subsequent downstream processing.

Bacillus subtilis

On the face of it, the Gram-positive organism *Bacillus subtilis*, seemed a more likely choice as a production organism. *B. subtilis* lacks the external lipopolysaccharide-rich membrane, alleviating endotoxin concerns, and easing protein secretion. In the event, production of albumin again proved too much for the bacterial system. Secretion of the protein was quite inefficient, probably not surprising in view of the fact that prokaryote and eukaryote secretion pathways are markedly different in a number of respects.

THE EUKARYOTES

Experience has taught us about the limitation of bacterial systems. Fortunately work with eukaryotes is proving rather less of a frustration. A number of eukarotic yeasts are being explored.

Kluyveromyces lactis

Kluyveromyces lactis is being developed by Gist Brocades and the organism, as the name suggests, can grow on lactose. The genetics of the organism are well understood and high levels of secretion of authentic human albumin are reportedly achieved.

Pichia pastoris

Phillips Petroleum are progressing *Pichia pastoris*, a methylotrophic yeast. The organism can be grown on methanol, again a cheap feedstock. In addition, a very powerful methanol oxidase promoter can give very high levels of recombinant protein synthesis.

Saccharomyces cerevisiae

Delta Biotechnology are concentrating their efforts on developing *Saccharomyces cerevisiae* as a process organism. To minimize costs, Delta's initial aim was to produce recombinant albumin (rHA) by exploiting the waste yeast recovered after the brewing of beer. Indeed, it was demonstrated that the albumin gene could be introduced into brewing yeast and by using a galactose-activated promoter, upstream of the gene, synthesis of albumin could be 'switched on' after beer production. Whilst the quality of the beer produced by the manipulated yeast was retained, there were a number of reasons why this process option was not progressed. It was recognized at a relatively early stage that the contribution of waste yeast to overall cost savings was minimal. Secondly, manipulation of the brewing yeast with a human gene posed significant regulatory problems. Thirdly, to ensure no leakage of human protein into the beer during fermentation, intracellular production of albumin was thought to be the necessary option. Unfortunately, intracellular production of albumin in *S. cerevisiae* is associated with the same problems as seen with *E. coli*. The N-terminal methionine is not cleaved and the protein is insoluble in the cell requiring renaturation.

It was calculated that on full-scale production, the urea requirement for solubilization of the cellular protein would involve the entire output of a medium-sized fertilizer plant. There is no doubt that disposal of the partially diluted and contaminated urea stream containing reductant would be environmentally hazardous.

The secretory pathway of a yeast, however, shares many features common to the higher eukaryotes and there was reason to believe that secretion of correctly folded protein with an authentic N-terminal could be achieved. This has in fact proved to be the case using a dedicated yeast system. The programme is being progressed in three main areas involving the development of an optimized production organism, fermentation conditions for growing the organism, and downstream processes for extraction and purification of the protein. Awareness of costs and regulatory issues have had a material impact on the development programme from the outset.

THE PRODUCTION ORGANISM

Vector systems for cloning in yeasts are most commonly based on the 2 μm plasmid, which is found in nearly all strains of *S. cerevisiae*. They have been chosen for this purpose because of their relatively high copy number and stability. In addition to the sequences for recombinant protein expression, there are minimum requirements for such plasmids. An *E. coli* origin of replication and a selectable marker, often for antibiotic resistance, are required for bacterial transformation. For yeast transformation, the requisites are a yeast origin of replication and a selectable marker, for example one which confers prototrophy for leucine. Finally, DNA sequences for stable replication are required.

With the basic DNA sequences in place to ensure plasmid maintenance, the albumin cDNA with suitable leader and promoter sequences, needs to be cloned into the vector. To secrete a heterologous protein, it is necessary to use a leader sequence which carries the appropriate signal sequences for directing a yeast protein out of the cell. Examples of such leader sequences are those directing secretion of invertase, phosphatase and α-mating factor (MFα1). Quite fortuitously it was found that albumin could be secreted from the yeast host using the natural albumin leader sequence. In practice, a hybrid leader, incorporating signal sequences from the natural albumin leader and MFα1, has proved optimal.

Having selected an appropriate leader sequence, a suitable promoter and transcription terminator are required upstream and downstream, respectively, of the coding region. The promoter may be either constitutive or inducible.

The major theoretical advantage of an inducible promotor is that production of any heterologous protein, even if it has no direct effect on the production organism, must to some extent be a drain on the cell's resources, and

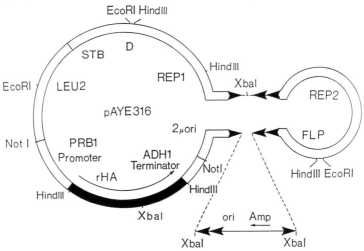

Fig. 9.6. A schematic representation of a disintegration vector. The figure shows the expression cassette for human albumin consisting of the structural gene, the promoter and terminator regions. The *Leu2* gene codes for a protein which enables the yeast to be grown selectively on a leucine-free substrate. The REP1, REP2, FLP, STB and ORI are DNA sequences required for stable replication

might be expected to lead to some reduction in yield or growth rate. The experience in bacterial systems is that this instability is so severe that the use of an inducible promoter is obligatory. In yeasts, however, the effect seems to be less severe, and a constitutive promoter can be used. Such an expression cassette, carried on a 2 μm plasmid, is extremely stable and lends itself to a large-scale production process. However, in practice, the large size of these plasmids renders them very difficult to manipulate. Delta has developed a system for manipulating these plasmids through the intermediary *E. coli*, subsequently introducing them into yeast where they spontaneously lose their *E. coli* DNA sequences.

The so-called 'disintegration' vector used for expressing human albumin, carries all the sequence necessary for independent replication, and has therefore proved to be quite exceptionally stable with no loss of plasmid observed over 300 generations. Plasmid stability in excess of 40 generations is an absolute requirement for a large-scale fermentation process (Figure 9.6).

FERMENTATION

The production of tens of tonnes of protein implies a fermentation capacity of hundreds or even thousands of tonnes of yeast per annum. In order to minimize the size and capital cost of the plant, intensive fermentation, operating at high final biomass is essential. The protein is secreted into the medium, which has imposed criteria on the selection of a feedstock. The feedstock needs to be cheap but it also needs to be defined and simple to minimize demands on downstream purification. The medium under development is composed of minimal salts, trace elements and vitamins. The nitrogen requirement is satisfied by using ammonia and the carbon source supplied by glucose or sucrose.

DOWNSTREAM PROCESSING

Due to the exceptionally high therapeutic dose of albumin, the necessity for very highly purified recombinant albumin is mandatory. The necessity to maximize purity without sacrificing yield imposes severe demands on downstream processing. The supernatant liquor, when separated from the cells, is enriched with the secreted albumin protein. Optimally the albumin is recovered by using a sequence of chromatographic separations followed by ultrafiltration.

REGULATORY ISSUES

Guidelines for developing biopharmaceutical products, using recombinant DNA technology, have been prepared by Regulatory authorities worldwide. However, it is constantly stressed that both the regulators and industry are on a learning curve and ultimately each potential product needs to be approached on a case by case basis.

There are a number of points to consider with regard to a recombinant albumin. Solutions of plasma-derived albumin have been used in clinical practice for some 40 years, hence if recombinant albumin is structurally identical, the therapeutic efficacy will not be in doubt. Clinical experience with HSA demonstrates that the protein is intrinsically 'not toxic' despite the high doses infused. A 10–12.5 g minimum dose of recombinant protein is, however, several orders of magnitude higher than any recombinant product developed to date. Expectations with regard to purity are consequently going to be high.

The production organism, *S. cerevisiae*, is non-pathogenic and man has been exposed to the organism very frequently through consumption of products such as bread and beer. Unlike *E. coli* or other Gram-negative bacteria, yeasts do not have endotoxin associated with the cell envelope. Essentially then, the recombinant protein must be shown to be structurally identical to the plasma protein, with process contaminants minimal and no toxicity.

In order to establish structural identity, it is important to have a standard preparation of plasma albumin with which to compare the recombinant protein. Unfortunately, albumin derived from large pools of donor plasma cannot be described as 'nature identical'. It is recovered from plasma by precipitation with high concentrations of alcohol and subsequently it is heat treated, at 60°C for 10 h, to kill viral contaminants. Also, binding sites of the protein are occupied by a variety of entities such as haem, bilirubin, fatty acids and often drugs like aspirin and penicillin. In the circumstances, an in-house standard has been carefully prepared, avoiding the pitfalls of the commercially fractioned product.

There are a number of tests which can be used to establish primary and tertiary structure of albumin. Very obviously, all the 585 amino acids can be sequenced. Such a task is not trivial and is certainly not routine. In any event, information confirming the primary sequence can be obtained indirectly on a more routine basis. Sequencing of the cDNA can be used to back-check on the protein sequence. Peptide mapping and amino acid analysis can be used routinely to verify the total amino acid profile.

Obviously it is important to confirm correct processing of the protein; the first 15 residues at the N-terminal and the last three residues at the C-terminal can be verified routinely. The N-terminal is a high-affinity binding site for copper, providing further evidence of authenticity.

A number of physico-chemical methods can be applied routinely. Gel filtration and SDS-PAGE are used to confirm molecular weight. Ion-exchange, chromatofocussing and isoelectric focussing are used to confirm charge. Ligand binding studies can provide confirmation of tertiary structure. Binding of fatty acids, bilirubin and some drugs can be measured

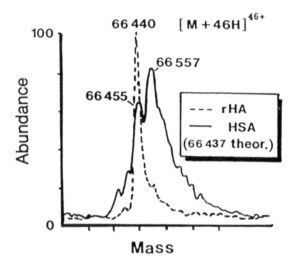

Fig. 9.7. Shows a comparison of rHA with HSA using electrospray mass spectroscopy. The spectra obtained show 'ion abundance' at different mass charge ratios

routinely. Rather less routinely, more sophisticated techniques, such as circular dichroism can be used to confirm helical content, X-ray crystallography and mass spectroscopy to confirm structure and molecular weight (Figure 9.7).

With regard to potential contaminants in the final product, as with the production of any biopharmaceutical, the development of a controlled production process using defined raw materials is paramount. This allows for early identification of potential product contaminants and development of sensitive assays to enable their detection and control. It is important to recognize that any definition of purity is only as good or even as bad, as the sensitivity of the assay concerned. Similarly, the definition of purity is only meaningful if it is qualified by an assessment of toxicity of a particular contaminant.

In summary, the overall objective is the production of tens of tonnes of recombinant albumin, at a competitive cost and sufficiently pure to allow a safe dosage of up to 150 g.

Because efficient productivity is only part of the challenge, for the production of human albumin, yeasts are proving to be very much more successful production organisms than bacteria. The scale of fermentation and the very large protein dose impose stringent criteria on organism stability, downstream processing, process validation and control throughout the production cycle.

Currently, although a recombinant human albumin has not yet been progressed through to clinical trial, there is no doubt that over the last few years there have been tremendous strides made toward meeting these objectives.

FURTHER READING

Advances in Blood Substitute Research: Proceedings of International Symposium, San Francisco, 1982. Progress in Clinical and Biological Research, **122**.

Arai, K., Ishioko, N., Huss, K., Madison, J. and Putnam, F.W. (1989) Identical structure changes in inherited albumin variants from different populations. *Proceedings of the National Academy of Science (USA),* **86**, 434–438.

Benesch, R. and Benesch, R.E. (1981) Preparation and properties of hemoglobin modified with derivatives of pyridoxal. *Methods in Enzymology,* **76**, 147–159.

Brown, J.R. (1977) Serum albumin: amino acid sequences. In: *Albumin Function and Uses.* Pergamon Press, Oxford.

Carter, D.C. *et al.* (1989) Three dimensional structure of human albumin. *Science,* **244**, 1195–1198.

Chinery, S.A. and Hincliffe, E. (1989) A novel class of vector for yeast transformation. *Current Genetics,* **61**, 21–25.

Kragh Hansen, U. (1981) Molecular aspects of ligand binding to serum albumin. *Pharmacological Reviews,* **33**(1), 17–53.

Latta, M. *et al.* (1989) Synthesis and purification of mature human serum albumin from *E. coli. Biotechnology,* **5**, 1309–1314.

Lawn, R.M. *et al.* (1981) The sequence of human serum albumin cDNA and its expression in *E. coli. Nucleic acid Research,* **922**, 6103–6114.

Lowe, K.C. (Ed.) (1988) *Blood Substitutes: Preparation, Physiology and Medical Applications.* Ellis-Horwood/VCH.

Rabinovici, R., Rudolph, A.S., Ligler, F.S., Yue, T.L. and Fuerstein, G. (1990) Liposome-encapsulated haemoglobin: an oxygen carrying fluid. *Circulatory Shock,* **32**, 1–17.

Savitsky, J.P., Doczi, J., Black, J. and Arnold, J.D. (1978) A clinical safety trial of stroma-free haemoglobin. *Clinical Pharmacology and Therapeutics,* **23**, 73–80.

Sehgal, L.R., Rosen, A.L., Gould, S.A., Sehgal, H.L., DeWoskin, R. and Moss, G.S. (1988) Hemoglobin solutions as red cell substitutes. *Progress in Transfusion Medicine,* **3** (Ed. J.D. Cash). Churchill Livingstone, Edinburgh.

Sleep, D., Belfield, G.P. and Goodey, A.R. (1990) The secretion of human serum albumin from the yeast *Saccharomyces cerevisiae* using five different leader sequences. *Biotechnology,* **8**, 42–46.

The Red Cell: 7th Ann Arbor Conference (1989) Progress in Clinical and Biological Research, **319**.

Tullis, J. (1977) Albumin. 1. Background and use. *Journal of the American Medical Association,* **237**(4), 355–360.

Tullis, J. (1977) Albumin. 2. Guidelines for clinical use. *Journal of the American Medical Association,* **237**(5), 460–463.

10 Cytokines and Growth Factors

H.A. LEAVER and P.L. YAP

Cytokines constitute a diverse group of protein molecules involved in inter-communication between cells involved in inflammation and immune responses and which also affect cell growth and function. The first important event in the identification of cytokines occurred in 1957 when Isaacs and Lindenmann reported a factor, which they called 'interferon', produced by cells in response to viral infections, and which could protect other cells of the same type from attack by a wide range of other viruses. For many years subsequently, the identification and investigation of cytokines was hampered by difficulties of assays and purification, but the last decade has seen an explosion in the knowledge of the structure and function of cytokines.

The identification of the various cytokines and peptide regulatory factors has paralleled developments in immunology, molecular biology and medicine and it is clear, in retrospect, that many individual biological factors previously described, were in fact one or more cytokines which have now been characterized. For instance, the factor which Isaacs and Lindenmann discovered in 1957, and which they called interferon is now known to encompass three different proteins (IFN-α, IFN-β and IFN-γ) with at least 16 additional subtypes of IFN-α. Many of the reports on the identification and characterization of cytokines based upon biological assays have now been superseded by the assay of molecular species using specific immunoassays, and pure standards, and by the analysis of specific mRNA sequences using hybridization techniques.

This brief review will describe the current knowledge of the structure and function of the various cytokines. In addition, because recombinant technology has allowed the manufacture of relatively large quantities of various cytokines such as IL-2 and IFN-α, some of the therapeutic applications will also be described. For more detailed information on cytokines, various articles in the Further Reading list should be consulted.

NOMENCLATURE AND GENERAL PROPERTIES OF CYTOKINES

Since the initial discoveries of various biological activities that are now attributed to cytokines, there have been a large number of reports on

Plasma and Recombinant Blood Products in Medical Therapy
Edited by C.V. Prowse. Published 1992 by John Wiley & Sons Ltd

Table 10.1 Nomenclature of some cytokines, with synonyms

Interleukin-1 α (IL-1α)	Lymphocyte activating factor (LAF)
Interleukin-1 β (IL-1β	Endogenous pyrogen (EP)
Interleukin-2 (IL-2)	T-cell growth factor (TCGF)
Interleukin-3 (IL-3)	Multi-colony stimulating factor (multi-CSF), mast-cell growth factor
Interleukin-4 (IL-4)	B-cell growth factor-1 (BCGF-1) B-cell stimulating factor-1 (BSF-1)
Interleukin-5 (IL-5)	Eosinophil differentiation factor (EDF) B-cell growth factor-II (BCGF-II)
Interleukin-6 (IL-6)	B-cell stimulating factor-2 (BSF-2) Interferon-β_2 (IFN-β_2) Hepatocyte stimulating factor (HSF)
Interleukin-7 (IL-7)	Lymphopoietin-1 (LP-1)
Interleukin-8 (IL-8)	Neutrophil activating factor (NAF) Monocyte-derived neutrophil activating protein (MONAP)
Tumour necrosis factor-α (TNF-α)	Cachectin
Tumour necrosis factor-β (TNF-β)	Lymphotoxin (LT)
Interferon-α (IFN-α)	Leukocyte interferon Acid-stable interferon Type-I interferon
Interferon-α (IFN-β)	Fibroblast interferon Acid-stable interferon Type-I interferon
Interferon-γ (IFN-γ)	Immune interferon Acid-labile interferon Type-II interferon Macrophage-activating factor (MAF)
Granulocyte-colony stimulating factor (G-CSF)	
Macrophage-colony stimulating factor (M-CSF)	Colony stimulating factor-1 (CSF-1)
Granulocyte-macrophage colony stimulating factor (GM-CSF)	Colony stimulating activator-granulocyte macrophage (CSA-GM)
Erythropoietin (EPO)	
Platelet-derived growth factor (PDGF)	
Nerve growth factor (NGF)	
Transforming growth factor-α (TGF-α)	
Transforming growth factor-β (TGF-β)	
Epidermal growth factor (EGF)	Urogastrone
Insulin growth factor-I (IGF-I)	Somatomedin-C
Insulin growth factor-II	

cytokines and growth factors, many of which are confusing, in relation to earlier papers. This is because the nomenclature has changed, with the isolation and identification of specific cytokines. This review will use the nomenclature and abbreviations shown in Table 10.1 throughout, but the reader should be aware that new cytokines are still being discovered and characterized. Thus activities previously attributed to one cytokine, e.g. B-cell growth factor (BCGF), may now be attributed to two separate cytokines, IL-4 and IL-6.

The term 'cytokine' is used generally to indicate a group of peptides with effects on cells of the immune system. However, there are a number of terms that describe molecules with similar properties such as 'lymphokines', 'interleukins' and 'growth factors'.

Cytokines may be defined as inducible proteins that exercise specific receptor-mediated effects on target cells and/or on the cytokine-producing cells themselves. *Lymphokines* are soluble mediators produced by lymphoid cells, acting on various target cells, whereas *monokines* are soluble mediators produced by monocytes/macrophages acting on similar or different target cells. *Interleukin* is a generic name for cytokines released by leukocytes which have specific effects on other leucocytes: thus lymphokines and monokines may be considered in general to be interleukins. However, cells other than leukocytes can produce cytokines (e.g. endothelial cells are important producers of polypeptide mediators that are involved in the differentiation and proliferation of T and B lymphocytes, and in the regulation of haematopoiesis). Thus not all cytokines can be considered to be interleukins, and the

Table 10.2 Growth factors that are cytokines

Factor	Cell source	Target cell
PDGF	Platelets Endothelial cells Placenta Some tumour cells	Smooth muscle Placental trophoblast Glial cells
NGF	Prostate gland Central nervous system Submaxillary gland	Sympathetic neurones Sensory neurones Receptors also present in many cells and tissues
TGF-α	Tumour cells Placenta Embryos	Various epithelial and mesenchymal cells

TGF-β	Platelets
	Bone
	Placenta
	Kidney
		Inhibition of proliferation of a
		  wide variety of cell types;
		  stimulation of cell
		  proliferation in some
		  mesenchymal tissues

IGF-I	Almost all tissues	Receptors very widespread

general term 'cytokines' is now preferred over earlier terms. One of the characteristics of cytokines is that they act as growth factors. Conversely, some growth factors may be considered to be cytokines and are produced by a variety of cell sources with a variety of targets cell (e.g. PDGF, NGF, TGF and IGF-1; Table 10.2). In addition, there is an overlap between the definition of cytokine, and that of a classical hormone, as in the case of erythropoietin and it is almost impossible to define cytokines precisely. However, although many of the characteristics of cytokines are similar to thsoe of 'classical' hormones, there are a few important differences.

- Cytokines are produced by specialized and non-specialized cells of many different tissues and organs and in general act locally. Hormones are produced only by specialized cells of the endocrine glands and act at a distance. However, if cytokines such as IL-6 are released into the circulation, they may also act at a distance from the cells that produce them
- Receptors for cytokines are found on many cell types whereas receptors for hormones are found on a limited number of target cell types
- Cytokines may be mitogenic *in vitro* unlike hormones which are rarely mitogenic
- Cytokines are usually large polypeptides, proteins or glycoproteins whereas hormones may consist of steroids, amino acid derivatives or polypeptides of various sizes and proteins

Thus the distinction between cytokines and hormones is, in some cases, very minor, and to some extent, dependent on terminology.

In summary, despite attempts to standardize the nomenclature, the terminology still remains confusing, since several cytokines either retain earlier names which reflect a description of their activity (e.g. tumour necrosis factor, interferon, colony-stimulating factor), or have had their names changed as they were identified (e.g. interleukin-2, formerly called T-cell growth factor; interleukin-1, formerly called endogenous pyrogen). Some of the previous names of various cytokines are shown in Table 10.1 and are occasionally still used (e.g. somatomedin C, cachectin, lymphotoxin).

STIMULI FOR CYTOKINE RELEASE AND CYTOKINE RECEPTORS

Numerous problems exist in the understanding of the stimuli for the secretory mechanisms of various cytokines and their subsequent actions on different target cells and tissues. Cytokines are usually produced transiently and locally in response to a specific stimulus and act on adjacent or nearby cells. The same cell type may produce different cytokines, but the same cytokine may be produced by different cell sources. Different stimuli may cause the release of the same cytokine, whereas single stimuli may cause the

CYTOKINES AND GROWTH FACTORS   187

Table 10.3 Some examples of problems in the analysis of cytokines

Single cell type secretes multiple cytokines	Macrophage	IL-1, TNF-α, IFN-α, PDGF, TGF-β, EPO, GM-CSF, G-CSF
	Endothelial cells	IL-1, IL-6, G-CSF, GM-CSF
Different cell sources for the same cytokine	IL-1	Monocytes/macrophages, neutrophils, fibroblasts, endothelial cells, dendritic cells, various tumour cell lines of different origins
	TNF	Monocytes/macrophages, T and B lymphocytes, mast cells, monocytic and T-cell lines
Different stimuli release the same cytokine	IL-1	Lipopolysaccharide, phorbol esters, muramyl dipeptide, calcium ionophore A23187, immune complexes
	TNF	Lipopolysaccharide, phorbol esters, cytokines (e.g. IL-2, IFN-γ) viruses (e.g. Sendai virus) immune complexes, cell-wall components of mycobacteria
An identical trigger may stimulate different cytokines	Lipopolysaccharide	IL-1, TNF
Cytokines are pleiotropic and pleiotypic	IL-1 and TNF	IL-1 and TNF induce endothelial leukocyte adhesion molecules
		IL-1 and TNF induce endothelial cell pro-coagulant production
		IL-1 and TNF induce respiratory burst in neutrophils and monocytes
		IL-1 and TNF induce the production of various enzymes by fibroblasts, synoviocytes and chondrocytes
An identical activity may be due to multiple different cytokines	Chemotaxis	IL-1, PDGF, GM-CSF, MDNCF*
	Cell proliferation	TNF-α, IL-1, PDGF, G-CSF, GM-CSF, EPO
	Inhibition of cell proliferation	TNF-α, IL-1, TGF-β, IFN-α, IFN-γ

* Macrophage-derived neutrophil chemotactic factor.

release of different cytokines. Cytokines may be pleiotropic, i.e. may have the same biological activity on different cell types, but may also be pleiotypic, i.e. may evoke different responses in different cell types. Finally, each identical biological activity may be produced by different cytokines. Some examples of these characteristics are shown in Table 10.3.

In considering the interaction of cytokines with their receptors, it should be noted that cytokines are extremely potent substances, generally acting at picomolar concentrations, indicating that cytokines exert their effects by binding to their cell-surface receptor with a high affinity. These cell-surface receptors are specific for each cytokine, or group of cytokines, and are relatively low in number (10–10000 per cell), although they may increase in response to various stimuli.

The glycosylation of the cytokine may be important for its binding to its specific receptor. Natural cytokines undergo extensive post-translational modifications including variable glycosylation, phosphorylation, sulphation, processing at N- or C-terminals and it is often not clear whether the natural state of the cytokine is in monomeric, dimeric or polymeric form. One example of a cytokine that shows heterogeneity in glycosylation is IFN-γ. Studies of cytokine–cell-surface receptor interactions have used recombinant cytokines derived from bacterial cells which are not glycosylated and such binding experiments therefore may not accurately reflect the interaction of the 'natural' cytokines with their corresponding receptor. However, despite differences in structure, it appears that certain of the recombinant cytokines (e.g. human recombinant IFN-γ derived from E. coli) appear to be fully biologically active.

It should also be noted that the response of target cells to a cytokine is dependent on the degree of expression of the cytokine receptor on the target cell (which may vary depending on previous stimuli), and on the nature of the link between the receptor and the different signal transduction pathways within the target cell.

Some of the human and mouse cytokine cell-surface receptors have been cloned and sequenced (e.g. receptors for IL-1, IL-2, IL-3, IL-4, IL-6, IFN-γ, GM-CSF, M-CSF and EPO), and have yielded important functional information. For instance, the IL-2 receptor consists of two subunits α and β. The α-subunit is a 55-kDa protein which binds IL-2 with low affinity. Interestingly, only 13 amino acids of the α-subunit extend into the cytoplasmic domain and it is therefore unable to transmit an intracellular signal following cytokine binding. In contrast the β-subunit of IL-2 is a 75-kDa protein, with a cytoplasmic domain of 286 amino acids and is probably the trigger of the IL-2 signal pathway. Interaction of the α- and β-subunits form the high-affinity IL-2 receptor but, as with the GM-CSF receptor (described below), further additional cell components may be involved.

High-affinity TNF receptors are present on a variety of cell types and are an example of the autocrine properties of cytokine receptors in that activated monocytes not only produce TNF but also express TNF receptors, which subsequently bind secreted TNF. The affinity and binding capacity of the TNF receptor can be down-regulated by activators of protein-kinase C and receptor-bound TNF is rapidly internalized and degraded intracellularly. The intracellular events beyond the binding of TNF (and other cytokines) are not well characterized but involve GTP binding proteins which interact with different signal transduction pathways (e.g. adenylate cyclase and phospholipase C).

The receptors for human IL-6 and GM-CSF have also been cloned and have relatively small cytoplasmic portions (80 and 54 amino acids out of a total of 449 and 400 amino acids, respectively). However, the human IFN-γ receptor has a large cytoplasmic domain (223 amino acids out of a total of 489) but by itself, cannot transduce a biological response, suggesting that additional components are required for signal transduction. Similarly, the human GM-CSF receptor, which has an extracellular domain of 297 amino acids, binds GM-CSF with only a low affinity, suggesting that additional sub-units or proteins are required for a high-affinity receptor.

The receptors for growth factors such as EGF, PDGF and IGF-1 have common structural features. These consist of a large extracellular growth-factor binding domain, a single cell membrane spanning domain and a large cytoplasmic domain with tyrosine kinase activity. Interestingly, the M-CSF receptor also has a cytoplasmic domain with tyrosine kinase activity, and the amino acid sequences of PDGF and M-CSF receptors are very similar, suggesting that these two receptors originated as a result of gene duplication. Other homologies may be observed when amino acid sequences of the various cloned cytokine receptors are compared; for example, an immuno-globulin-like sequence can be found in the IL-1, IL-6 and IFN-γ receptors, and a weak but significant homology is observed for the IL-2β chain, the IL-3, IL-4 and IL-6 receptors, the EPO receptor and GM-CSF receptor.

These structure–function relationships, together with other evidence such as the weak homology with the prolactin receptor and growth-hormone receptor, suggest that many of the cytokine cell-surface receptors belong to the same supergene family and may originate from a single ancestral cell-surface receptor protein. The conservation of the structural region(s) of cytokine receptors involved in signal transduction indicate a restricted range of conformations in the regions interacting with similar proteins which transduce the signal into the cell interior. This hypothesis may also explain how a range of biological activities may be elicited by slightly different cytokines in different cell types, as triggering of similar cytokine receptors may be linked to different signal transduction pathways. This hypothesis may also explain how a range of biological activities may be elicited by the same cytokine in different cell types via receptors with varying conformations in the region which interacts with different cell signalling molecules.

SOME IMPORTANT CYTOKINES

IL-1

IL-1 is a multifunctional cytokine responsible for mediating a variety of processes in response to infection, inflammation and injury. Although originally identified as a fever-producing substance from neutrophils, and also as an endogenous pyrogen (EP), that could be isolated from the blood of rabbits receiving injections of bacteria or endotoxin. It was initially considered to be a co-factor for lymphocyte proliferation. IL-1 is now known to be produced by a variety of cell types and has many different target calls (Table 10.3). There are two genes producing two distinct but related molecules, IL-1 α and IL-1 β. Interestingly, although human and mouse IL-1 α are 62% homologous with each other, human IL-1 α and IL-1 β only show 26% homology. In most human tissues, IL-1β mRNA predominates over IL-1 α mRNA.

IL-1 α and IL-1 β bind to the same receptor, despite differences in the amino acid sequences, and it appears that neither form of IL-1 is glycosylated. Both proteins are available in recombinant form.

IL-1 has a variety of effects including the promotion of antigen-specific immune responses by the activation of T lymphocytes. It augments the production of IL-2 and induces the expression of IL-2 receptor on antigen-activated T-lymphocytes via the T-cell receptor, resulting in a rapid proliferation of such stimulated T lymphocytes. In addition, IL-1 appears to interact with IL-4 in B-lymphocyte activation and may also induce IL-6 in other cells, which in turn stimulates the differentiation of B lymphocytes.

IL-1 has an important role in acute inflammation and induces the production of prostaglandin E_2, collagenase and phospholipase A_2. IL-1 also appears to induce IL-6 production in cell types other than B lymphocytes, which results in other growth factors being produced, and IL-1 can also act as a stimulatory factor for hepatocytes to induce the production of many acute phase proteins. Thus IL-1 plays a pivotal role in inflammation.

IL-2

IL-2 was originally described as a T-cell growth factor produced by antigen- or mitogen-stimulated lymphocytes. The gene for IL-2 has been identified and cloned and recombinant IL-2 produced from bacteria, yeast, insect and mammalian cells. Naturally occurring IL-2 is glycosylated, but the carbohydrate groups do not appear to be important for its biological activity. Most IL-2 is secreted by helper T lymphocytes after stimulation by antigen binding to the T-cell receptor.

The binding of IL-2 to its receptor on T lymphocytes results in proliferation, increased secretion of other cytokines, increased expression of cell-surface receptors for other growth factors and also of major histocom-patibility complex (MHC) Class II molecules. In addition to the binding of IL-2 to mature T lymphocytes and thymocytes, IL-2 induces T-lymphocyte cytotoxicity and stimulates natural killer-cell activity. B lymphocytes may also be stimulated by IL-2. As with TNF, IL-2 acts as an autocrine growth factor, i.e. T lymphocytes secreting IL-2 express IL-2 receptors.

IL-3

IL-3 is produced by T lymphocytes and stimulates the growth and dif-ferentiation of pluripotent haematopoietic stem cells, leading to the pro-duction of the different blood cell types. This cytokine had different names previously (see Table 10.1) and it appears that IL-3 acts on the early stages of the development of haematopoietic cells. IL-3 and GM-CSF have many similar biological activities, but only IL-3 is able to stimulate mast-cell proliferation. IL-3 appears to act with other cytokines such as G-CSF and EPO in the full development of cells of the neutrophil or erythroid lineage, respectively.

IL-4

IL-4 was discovered as a factor that stimulated B lymphocytes to proliferate, but more recent evidence suggests that IL-4 may act as a growth factor for T lymphocytes. IL-4 has various effects on B lymphocytes: it induces produc-tion of IgE, causes isotype switching to IgG and induces the expression of MHC class II molecules. It is therefore important in the humoral immune response.

IL-4 can also stimulate the growth of mast cells and may act together with colony-stimulating factors to promote the growth of haematopoietic stem cells. IL-4 may have an effect on macrophages, similar to macrophage activa-tion factor (MAF) and can also stimulate the fusion of macrophages to form giant multi-nucleated cells. It has therefore been postulated that IL-4 may be involved in the development of the granulomatous response.

IL-5

IL-5 was first identified as a T-lymphocyte product that induced B lympho-cytes to differentiate into immunoglobulin-secreting cells after stimulation by antigen, and was called B-cell growth factor. IL-5 acts with IL-4 to regu-late the proliferation and differentiation of B lymphocytes. In addition, IL-5 appears to act as a eosinophil colony-stimulating and differentiating factor. Most of the information on IL-5 has been obtained using mouse IL-5 but human recombinant IL-5 has been shown to have several effects on B lym-phocytes, including the induction of IgM and IgA production.

IL-6

IL-6 is a multifunctional cytokine that mediates different host responses and regulates the development of multiple cell types. It is a differentiation factor for B lymphocytes, cytotoxic T lymphocytes and for haematopoiesis. The biological activities of IL-6 overlap with those of IL-1 and some of the pleiotropic effects of IL-1 are actually caused by IL-6 or by synergistic actions of IL-1 and IL-6. IL-6 stimulates hepatic protein synthesis during the acute-phase response and can act as an endogenous pyrogen. Interestingly, the gene for IL-6 is similar to that for G-CSF suggesting that these two genes originated from a common ancestral gene.

   IL-6 can be secreted by many cells, including T lymphocytes, monocytes/ macrophages, endothelial cells and fibroblasts and is released by damaged tissues. Plasma IL-6 levels in patients with sepsis are markedly increased and IL-6 has therefore been considered to be an 'alarm hormone' as it is involved in the systemic changes that are associated with infection and tissue injury.

IL-7

IL-7 was identified in studies of the long-term culture of bone marrow, and appears to be a growth factor for pre-B cells and for early development of the T-lymphocyte lineage. It does not appear to have any effect on mature B lymphocytes. In addition, IL-7 appears to be a growth factor for immature as well as adult thymocytes and mature T lymphocytes proliferate in response to IL-7. Thus IL-7 appears to be an important developmental factor for both T and B lymphocytes, but so far only the stromal cells from bone marrow and thymus have been shown to produce IL-7. There is no evidence that IL-7 has any effect on the proliferation and differentiation of any of the other haematopoietic cell lineage and IL-7 can therefore be considered to be a lymphoid specific regulator.

TNF

The action of a 'tumour necrotizing factor' was first described in 1962 in the serum of mice challenged with lipopolysaccharide (LPS) obtained from *Serratia marcescens*. In 1975, a similar activity was found in the serum of rodents and rabbits primed with Bacillus Calmette-Guerin (BCG), then challenged with LPS. This factor caused regression of some transplanted tumours *in vivo*, and was cytostatic or cytocidal to some tumour cells in culture, but did not affect normal human fibroblasts. The mediator, which was thought to originate from macrophages, was called 'tumour necrosis factor', but was also subsequently identified as chachectin.

   Two forms of TNF have now been identified: TNF-α or cachectin and TNF-β or lymphotoxin. TNF-α is secreted by activated macrophages, activated by LPS and other stimuli (Table 10.3) but is also secreted by activated natural-killer (NK) cells, T lymphocytes, fibroblasts and mast cells. TNF-β is secreted by lymphoblastoid cells, and antigen or mitogen-activated T lymphocytes. TNF-α and TNF-β are the product of two different genes and have only approximately 30% amino acid homology. Despite this, they have similar functions and both forms have a wide range of effects on neutrophils including an increase in neutrophil numbers, after *in vivo* administration (in rats), an accumulation of neutrophils at intradermal sites of injection (in rabbits), and an increased expression of surface adherence proteins and an increase in phagocytic activity. Recombinant human TNF-α has a weak but direct stimulus on neutrophil superoxide anion production, H_2O_2 production and myeloperoxidase–H_2O_2–halide activity.

The anti-tumour effect of TNF has been well characterized, although the exact mechanisms by which both forms of TNF mediate cytoxicity have not been identified. It is possible that the activation of neutrophils and their increased adherence to vascular endothelial cells, following TNF stimulation may in part explain the haemorrhagic necrosis of solid tumours and the associated inflammation.

TNF induces fever, initially by increasing prostaglandin E_2 synthesis in the hypothalamus and, subsequently, by triggering the production of IL-1. TNF also stimulates the release of other cytokines and factors, such as haematopoietic growth factors (G-CSF, GM-CSF), PDGF, platelet activating factor, prostacyclin and osteoclast activating factor. TNF has been implicated in the remodelling of connective tissue through an action on fibroblasts. TNF also appears to have a primary role as a mediator of septic shock, possibly following stimulation of monocytes/macrophages by LPS.

TNF has been implicated in the pathogenesis of the cachexia (anorexia, weight loss, anaemia, and depletion of whole-body protein and lipid) associated with chronic human diseases, but its exact role remains to be determined due to difficulties in the detection of TNF in the plasma of cachectic patients. However, animals chronically exposed to sublethal doses of TNF become cachectic and the derangements of lipid and protein metabolism induced by TNF resemble the metabolic alterations associated with injury, illness and bacterial infection.

THE INTERFERONS

Interferon (IFN) was originally discovered as an antiviral protein but there now appear to be several types of IFN and other biological effects extending beyond the antiviral effects. Interferons may be defined as proteins which exert non-specific antiviral activity, at least in homologous cells, through cellular metabolic processes involving synthesis of RNA and protein.

There are three main types of IFN and their properties are given in Table 10.4. There appear to be as many as 23 different human IFN-α genes and

Table 10.4 Properties of the interferons

Property	IFN-α	IFN-β	IFN-γ
Previous name	Leukocyte IFN	Fibroblast IFN	Immune IFN
Subtypes	At least 16	β_1 and β_2*	No subtypes
Main source	Null lymphocytes Monocytes Macrophages	Fibroblasts Epithelial cells	T lymphocytes NK cells
Main stimuli	Viruses Virally infected cells	Viruses Polynucleotides	Allogeneic cells, virally infected syngeneic cells, foreign antigens, T-cell mitogens
Location of gene	Chromosome 9	Chromosome 9	Chromosome 12
Homology	30% with β	30% with α	10% with α and β
Molecular weight	20 kDa	26 kDa	17 kDa
Amino acids	165	166	143–146
Glycosylation†	+	++	+++
Acid stability	Yes	Yes	No

* IFN-β_2 is now called 'IL-6' and shows a distant evolutionary relationship with IFN-α and IFN-β.
† –, +, ++, +++ denote increasing levels of glycosylation.

pseudogenes, giving rise to at least 16 closely related proteins known as 'sub-types'. It is not clear why there are so many subtypes of IFN-α, when there is only one IFN-β gene. There are few functional differences between the α subtypes and the clinical activity of individual α subtypes and naturally produced mixtures is identical. IFN-α is mainly produced by peripheral blood mononuclear cells and IFN-β by fibroblasts and epithelial cells. IFN-α production is stimulated by viruses, bacteria, xenogeneic or allogeneic tumour cells, virally infected cells and B-lymphocyte mitogens, while IFN-β production is stimulated by viruses and polynucleotides. IFN-γ is mainly secreted by activated T lymphocytes, in response to antigen or mitogen and can be distinguished by its lability to extremes of temperature or pH.

Although only limited information is available concerning the precise signals that are transmitted to the nucleus following the binding of IFN to the cell-surface receptor, it has been suggested that the inositol pathway is involved. Whatever the mechanism, the result is the up-regulation of some cellular genes, and the down-regulation of others. Interferons induce the expression of MHC class I genes, and in addition, IFN-γ activates class II MHC genes. Interferons also induce two enzymes that inhibit protein translation (2–5A synthetase and protein kinase) that are implicated in the anti-viral activity of this cytokine. In addition, the interferons have a multiplicity of effects on immune regulation, cell growth and differentiation and against tumours, which are summarized in Table 10.5.

Table 10.5 Actions of interferon

Action	IFN-α	IFN-β	IFN-γ
Induction of antiviral state	Yes	Yes	Yes
Induction of MHC Class I expression	Yes	Yes	Yes
Induction of MHC Class II	No	No	Yes
B-cell activation	–*	–	Yes
B-cell proliferation	No	–	–
B-cell differentiation	–	–	Yes
T-cell growth stimulation	–	–	Yes
Cytotoxic effects	Yes	–	Yes
Cytostatic effects	Yes	Yes	Yes
Antitumour activity *in vivo*	Yes	Yes	Yes
Fever Induction	Yes	Yes	Yes

* – indicates not known.

HAEMATOPOIETIC GROWTH FACTORS

The haematopoietic growth factors are cytokines that regulate the proliferation and differentiation of haematopoietic progenitor cells and the function of mature blood cells. The factors that have so far been identified and cloned consist of multi-CSF or IL-3, GM-CSF, G-CSF, M-CSF and erythropoietin (EPO). IL-3 has already been described. The haematopoietic growth factors interact with the various lineages of bone-marrow cells at different stages ranging from the multipotent progenitor cell to the circulating mature cell. These growth factors differ in molecular weight, chromosomal location, cellular source and target-cell lineage affected (Table 10.6) although the genes for GM-CSF, IL-3 and M-CSF are clustered on the same chromosome.

Table 10.6 Properties of haematopoietic growth factors

Factor	MW×10³ (kDa)	Cellular source	Target lineage
Multi-CSF (IL-3)	15–30	T lymphocytes	All lineages
GM-CSF	18–30	T lymphocytes Monocytes Fibroblasts Endothelial cells	Granulocytes Eosinophils Monocytes
G-CSF	20	Monocytes Fibroblasts Epithelial cells	Granulocytes
M-CSF	70–90	Monocytes Fibroblasts Endothelial cells	Monocytes
EPO	39	Peritubular cells of the kidney Kupffer cells	Erythrocyte

The production of growth factors by the various cell types (Table 10.6) is normally low but following stimulation with bacterial endotoxin (for monocytes) or foreign antigens (for T lymphocytes), levels can rise rapidly. An indirect stimulus may occur via IL-1, which is a potent inducer of haematopoietic growth factors.

The action of these growth factors is restricted to local areas adjacent to the sites of production and the distribution of specific cell-surface receptors for each growth factor. Development of the cell lineages may involve the action of one or more of the growth factors, for instance the production of megakaryocytes involves EPO interacting with IL-3, GM-CSF, IL-1 and thrombocytopoiesis-stimulating factor. Some factors are early acting, such as IL-3 and GM-CSF, whereas others are mainly late acting, such as EPO, G-CSF and M-CSF. In addition, other cytokines such as IL-4 and IL-5 are involved in the development of eosinophils.

Haematopoietic growth factors have functions other than the development of bone-marrow cells. GM-CSF sustains the viability and potentiates functions of phagocytic cells such as microbial killing, tumoricidal activity and the production of other cytokines. GM-CSF is a potent inhibitor of neutrophil migration and is therefore important in areas of infection and inflammation. G-CSF potentiates the survival and various functions of mature neutrophils and M-CSF enhances the production of various cytokines by monocytes and increases their tumoricidal activity.

CYTOKINE NETWORKS

From the preceding description of the properties of the different individual cytokines, it is clear that although individual cytokines have multiple overlapping cell regulatory activities, in general, cytokines interact in a coordinated or sequential fashion. An example of this is in the development of the various bone-marrow lineages, where certain cytokines act at the earlier stages of development and others act at later stages. This interaction has been called the 'cytokine network' and a detailed understanding of it is required if cytokines are to be used effectively in the therapy of human disease.

THE ROLE OF CYTOKINES IN INFLAMMATION

IL-1 is one of the main cytokines involved in inflammation, by increasing vascular permeability, possibly through PGE_2 release from different cell types in connective tissue. As described earlier, IL-1 and TNF are also involved in an alteration of the vascular adherence of leukocytes, induction of endothelial cell pro-coagulant production and an alteration in bacterial killing. Furthermore, IL-1 and TNF also induce production of prostacyclin and platelet activating factor (PAF). PAF is of particular importance since it may be responsible for part of the hypotension and shock induced by endotoxin, as well as the increased permeability of the vascular endothelium that occurs in acute inflammation.

The term 'acute phase response' is used to describe the range of host humoral and cellular responses to severe system injury or infection. IL-1, TNF and IL-6 are important cytokines mediating the acute-phase response and are mainly released by monocytes/macrophages in response to various harmful stimuli. As stated earlier, IL-6 is of particular importance since it was shown to be identical to the hepatocyte stimulating factor which stimulates the liver to produce the major acute phase proteins.

Finally, the recovery from inflammation involves tissue remodelling. IL-1 and IL-6 are involved in protease production, and induce the production of various enzymes such as collagenase and gelatinase from cells such as fibroblasts, synoviocytes and chondrocytes. TNF and IL-1 also induce fibroblast and mesenchymal cell proliferation, and growth factors such as TGF-β. IL-1β has been shown to be identical to osteoclast-activating factor, which induces osteoclast bone-resorbing activity, and TNF and IL-1 inhibit synthesis of proteoglycan, an essential component of cartilage as well as stimulating cartilage resorption.

THE ROLE OF CYTOKINES IN THE IMMUNE RESPONSE

The main cytokines involved in the development of an immune response are IL-1, IL-2, IL-4 and IL-6. IL-2 and IL-4 act as T-lymphocyte growth factors whereas IL-1 enhances T-lymphocyte proliferation. On its own, IL-1 is a poor stimulator of T-lymphocyte proliferation, but has a synergistic effect, in combination with antigen or lectin mitogens. It has also been suggested that IL-1 may be active in a membrane-bound form on the surface of accessory cell such as monocytes/macrophages, since addition of neutralizing IL-1 antibodies to lymphocytes and monocytes had no effect on antigen- or mitogen-stimulated T-lymphocyte proliferation. Whatever the mechanism, IL-1 induces the production of IL-2 and other cytokines, such as IL-3, IL-4, IL-5, IL-6, IL-7, GM-CSF, TNF-α, and TGF-β which may be produced by activated T lymphocytes.

IL-6 is also important in the early stages of the immune response. Resting T lymphocytes express high-affinity receptors for IL-6 and it is possible that IL-6 may be responsible for some of the accessory cell activity not attributable to IL-1, described above. IL-6 also acts as a differentiation factor for cytotoxic T lymphocytes, and stimulates the proliferation of thymocytes.

Cytokines are also important in the development of B lymphocytes. IL-7, thought to derive from bone-marrow stromal cells appears to stimulate early development and proliferation of B lymphocytes. Other cytokines, such as IL-1, IL-3 and IL-4 augment B lymphocyte proliferation and differentiation during episodes of infection. IL-4, IL-5 and IFN-γ may also be involved in the switching of immunoglobulin isotypes, i.e. the sequential secretion of different isotypes of immunoglobulin with the same specificity, during the development of a specific antibody response.

CYTOKINES FOR THERAPY

As cytokines appear to be involved in the host response to many disease processes, there has been a great deal of research on therapeutic applications. However, in considering current therapeutic approaches, a number of caveats are necessary:

- The role of cytokines in health and disease is complex and augmenting or decreasing specific cytokine levels may not be easily achieved, or effective in disease treatment
- Cytokines are produced locally, released into micro-environments and act on adjacent cells. Systemically administered cytokines may not reach target micro-environments
- Many cell types have cytokine receptors: target-cell specificity of cytokines is usually limited

Table 10.7 Cytokines for therapeutic use

Cytokine	Product	Application
IL-1	Recombinant IL-1α Recombinant IL-1β	Antitumour
IL-2	Recombinant IL-2	Antitumour Antibacterial
IL-3	Recombinant IL-3	Stem-cell survival and restoration of leukocytes following chemotherapy
IL-4	Recombinant IL-4	Antitumour
IFN-α	Leukocyte IFN Lymphoblastoid IFN Recombinant IFN-α	Antitumour Antiviral
IFN-A	Fibroblast IFN-β Recombinant IFN-β	Antitumour Antiviral
IFN-γ	Recombinant IFN-γ	Antitumour Chronic granulomatous disease Rheumatoid arthritis
G-CSF	Recombinant G-CSF	Restoration of leukocyte count after chemotherapy or marrow transplantation
GM-CSF	Recombinant GM-CSF	Restoration of leukocyte count after chemotherapy or bone-marrow transplantation
TNF-α	Recombinant TNF-α	Antitumour
EPO	Recombinant EPO	Anaemia of chronic renal failure

- Some cytokines have very short half-lives *in vivo*, thus repeated therapy may be necessary
- Some cytokines may be very toxic in therapeutic doses. This is particularly true of systemically administered cytokines which may have to be administered in large doses to reach the desired site of action

A summary of the cytokines that are currently in use or in clinical trials is shown in Table 10.7 and some of the therapeutic applications of individual cytokines such as IL-2, TNF, IFN-α, and the haematopoietic growth factors will be considered in more detail.

SPECIFIC CYTOKINES

IL-1

IL-1 is produced by almost every nucleated cell type in response to injury, as well as by monocytes and macrophages during the immune response. However, due to its wide range of activities, it is too non-specific for therapeutic use and may have serious toxicity.

Nonetheless, IL-1 has been shown to be associated with tumour regression in mice, following intra-lesional injection, and also to enhance the resistance of normal and neutropenic mice to *Pseudomonas* and *Klebsiella* infection. Thus, IL-1 may have a potential role as an anti-tumour agent or in the treatment of infection.

IL-2

IL-2 is the most important T-cell growth factor, and mononuclear cells exposed to IL-2 develop cytotoxic reactivity against autologous and allogeneic tumour cells. Treatment of mice with recombinant IL-2 or recombinant IL-2 activated T lymphocytes can produce a partial remission of liver and lung metastases. Clinical trials have therefore been performed in patients with various malignancies, with a beneficial response occurring in some patients. However, the severe toxic effects of IL-2 therapy have been a major problem (see below) and two main approaches have been used in current trials of IL-2 therapy:

(1) Instead of intermittent administration of large doses of IL-2, lower doses have been administered by continuous infusion. As a result of such therapy, similar clinical responses to IL-2 to high-dose IL-2 therapy, but with reduced toxicity was seen in patients with a wide range of malignancies such as malignant melanoma, renal, ovarian, lung and parotid cancer, and Hodgkin's disease and malignant lymphoma.

(2) Adoptive IL-2 immunotherapy using lymphokine-activated killer (LAK) cells has been extensively investigated. This treatment involves obtaining

lymphocytes from cancer patients by repeated leukaphereses, incubating the cells with IL-2 *in vitro* to generate LAK cells, and re-infusing the LAK cells in conjunction with IL-2. Patients with renal cell cancer, malignant melanoma, non-Hodgkin's lymphoma and rectal cancer have shown complete responses to such a therapeutic approach, although in these studies, severe IL-2 or LAK cell-associated toxicity was observed in some patients and treatment schedules.

IL-2 therefore appears to be a promising anti-cancer agent, but clearly further clinical studies are required to increase the therapeutic effect, since many patients do not respond, or only show minor or partial responses. This may involve modification of dose, treatment schedules and numbers of treatment courses. When LAK cells are used, methods of increasing the potency of the cells cytotoxic to tumours is required. Finally, IL-2 therapy, like other forms of cytokine therapy remains very expensive.

TNF

TNF has an anti-tumour activity in some animal models, and some tumour lines *in vitro*, and TNF has therefore been explored as an anti-tumour agent. Although Phase I and early Phase II studies have been performed in many hundreds of patients with disseminated cancers refractory to conventional therapy, only sporadic patients with tumour regression have been reported. However, some of the individual case reports suggest that TNF may still be a promising form of therapy. For example, a patient with a soft-tissue sarcoma, developed haemorrhagic necrosis of his tumour following TNF therapy. In addition, results of studies using intra-lesional or intraperitoneal administration of TNF have shown more promising results, with one patient with a neuroendocrine tumour showing a complete remission following TNF therapy.

Current clinical studies are therefore focussed on the combination of TNF with other cytokines such as IL-2 and the interferons. This approach is logical, as cytokines act either sequentially or synergistically, and two patients with chronic myeloid leukaemia, who were refractory to IFN-α therapy, responded to a combination of IFN-α with TNF. In addition, another approach may be to use TNF in the generation of LAK cells (described above) since synergism occurs between TNF and IL-2 in this process. Finally, it is possible that better results may be obtained in cancer patients if TNF is used together with existing chemotherapy agents or at an earlier stage of the malignancy.

Interferons

In the 1970s, the interferons were heralded as a major breakthrough in cancer therapy. However, despite numerous clinical studies, and a major investment in the production of non-recombinant IFN-α and IFN-β, inter-feron therapy has only been licensed for a very small number of conditions. More recently, the availability of recombinant IFN-α has resulted in an increase in the number of diseases in which the effects of IFN therapy has been investigated.

IFN-α in therapy of cancer and viral infections

The use of IFN-α has been investigated in a large number of malignancies but only hairy-cell leukaemia is highly responsive. Other haematological malignancies that are partially responsive include non-Hodgkin's lym-phoma, chronic granulocytic leukaemia, essential thrombocythaemia and cutaneous T-cell lymphoma. Among the solid tumours, complete or partial responses have been seen in IFN-α therapy for Kaposi's sarcoma (AIDS related), melanoma, renal cell, ovarian and head-and-neck (squamous) cancer, and some bladder cancers. However, the response rate with com-monly occurring cancers such as breast, lung and colorectal cancers has been very disappointing. Furthermore, most of the evidence so far indi-cates that IFN-α is not beneficial when used together with conventional anti-cancer chemotherapy. Toxicity, as with IL-2 therapy, has been a prob-lem when higher doses have been used, and in general, relatively low doses are now used.

Interferon was first described as an antiviral agent and it is not surprising that IFN-α and IFN-β have been extensively investigated in various viral infections. IFN-α, administered as an intra-nasal spray can prevent, but not cure, rhinovirus infections. However, although this virus accounts for 40% of 'common colds', the side-effects from repeated spraying, such as stuffi-ness and nasal erosions, prevent the widespread use of IFN-α for this indica-tion. Human papilloma virus is associated with recurrent laryngeal papillomatosis and condylomata acuminata, and intra-lesional or intra-muscular IFN-α therapy in such conditions has shown very encouraging results. Furthermore, the topical application of IFN-α as a cream or ointment to lesions of genital herpes has a limited beneficial effect.

Some patients with chronic hepatitis B, hepatitis C or non-A,non-B hepa-titis infection develop cirrhosis and hepatocellular carcinoma. Many pro-spective trials have been undertaken with IFN-α in such patients and, in some recipients, the hepatitis resolves with a reduction, in the case of chronic hepatitis B, of HBe antigenaemia and HBV DNA levels. Unfor-tunately, in a few of the responders, hepatitis B viral re-activation occurs on cessation of IFN-α therapy, except in those responders who no longer express HBV sequences in their genome. The inability to predict which patients are likely to respond and the cost and side-effects of long-term IFN-α therapy suggest that the widespread use of IFN-α in the treatment of chronic hepatitis is unlikely.

IFN-β has, in general, been shown to have similar results to IFN-α in the treatment of virally mediated diseases. However, when IFN-β is administered by intramuscular injection, it tends to remain localized, whereas IFN-α enters the circulation quickly. More recently, recombinant IFN-γ has become available for clinical trials but preliminary reports have not been very encouraging. IFN-γ has not been effective in the treatment of solid tumours although there may be a possible benefit in lymphoproliferative diseases. Interestingly, preliminary data suggest that IFN-γ may have a role in autoimmune diseases. In rheumatoid arthritis, disease remissions have been recorded, and a beneficial effect in the rare congenital disorder, chronic granulomatosis disease has also been reported.

Haemopoietic growth factors

Many cytokines are involved in the development of the various cell lineages in the bone marrow (see above), and several of the haematopoietic growth factors have now been tested in a variety of clinical trials. Erythropoietin (EPO) has been shown to have a beneficial effect on haematocrit and reticulocyte counts in patients with anaemia associated with chronic renal failure, and in such patients, the transfusion requirements have been greatly reduced. Concomitant with the increase in haemoglobin level have been subjective improvements in appetite, energy and exercise tolerance. However thromboses, hypertension and stroke have been reported following increases in blood viscosity after EPO treatment, but the adverse effects other than hypertension can be reduced by gradual administration of EPO so that the haematocrit only rises slowly. Some of the other forms of anaemia have also been investigated with EPO. The anaemia accompanying zidovudine therapy in human immunodeficiency virus (HIV) infected patients has been shown to be responsive to EPO therapy as has the anaemia associated with rheumatoid arthritis. Unfortunately, the cost of EPO therapy at present is likely to prevent widespread use of EPO in patients with conditions other than the severe anaemia associated with chronic renal failure.

G-CSF has been shown to increase neutrophil counts in a dose-related manner, as long as G-CSF treatment is being administered. However, neutrophil counts fall to pretreatment levels within a few days of cessation of therapy. GM-CSF produces similar rises in neutrophil, monocyte and eosinophil counts but it appears that GM-CSF is slightly less effective than G-CSF in raising leukocyte counts, and high doses of GM-CSF are also associated with toxicity, unlike G-CSF. Thus the therapeutic role of G-CSF and GM-CSF is likely to be in raising leukocyte counts after chemotherapy, or bone-marrow transplantation and also possibly in patients with aplastic anaemia or AIDS-related leukopenia. However, in patients with AIDS, GM-CSF may enhance infection with HIV, since monocytes are an important reservoir for infection with this virus, and GM-CSF may need to be administered with antiretroviral drugs. Patients with myelodysplastic disorders may also benefit from GM-CSF or G-CSF therapy but caution is required in these diseases, since such growth factors have been shown to induce a proliferative response in leukaemic cells. Furthermore, as the myelodysplastic diseases are chronic, repeated life-long administration of a short-acting drug would be required.

SIDE-EFFECTS OF CYTOKINE THERAPY

Multiple serious side-effects have been observed with cytokine therapy. For instance, fever, fatigue, anaemia, hypoalbuminaemia, eosinophilia, rashes, nausea, diarrhoea, weight gain, dyspnoea, hypotension, tachyarrhythmia and congestive heart failure have been recorded with recombinant IL-2 therapy and LAK cell therapy.

With IFN-α therapy, an acute syndrome of fever, chills and influenza-like symptoms occurs within hours of commencing such therapy, although such symptoms tend to be self-limiting and tolerance develops within a week or so. The symptoms appear to be a direct effect of IFN-α itself, rather than due to a contaminant of the IFN-α preparation and fatigue is the most frequent dose-limiting side-effect. In general, most treatment schedules with IFN-α aim to use relatively low doses (e.g. 3 million units three times a week administered subcutaneously with simultaneous administration of paracetamol to reduce the side-effects).

G-CSF is tolerated well although both GM-CSF and G-CSF have been associated with bone-pain, and with transient leukopenia in the first half-hour after intravenous bolus injection. The transient leukopenia is not associated with any untoward clinical effects. In contrast to G-CSF, GM-CSF is associated with fever, malaise, myalgia, arthralgia, anorexia, mild elevations in transaminase levels and a rash localized to the site of the injection. At higher doses of GM-CSF, more serious side-effects consisting of a capillary leak syndrome and large-vessel thrombosis have been observed, whereas no comparable maximal tolerated dose has been defined for G-CSF.

FUTURE DEVELOPMENTS IN CYTOKINE THERAPY

In view of the severe toxicity associated with some of the cytokines, alternative approaches to cytokine therapy have been used. For instance, cytokines can be 'targetted' to certain tissues only, by conjugation with monoclonal antibodies. Such conjugates would reduce the dose of cytokine needed with reduced toxicity and possibly result in a longer half-life in the target tissue. Such an approach has been demonstrated for IFN-α conjugated to monoclonal antibodies, and these conjugates have an enhanced anti-proliferative action, compared with IFN-α alone. Hybrid proteins, such as that recently described for IFN-γ and TNF-β have also been constructed, and combination of the active portion of cytokines to other proteins, using recombinant technology, is likely to be an increasingly attractive approach.

Another approach has been to identify natural inhibitors of the cytokines. IL-1 inhibitory activities have been observed in human fluids, and in the supernatants of cultured human or animal cells or cell lines, and an IL-1 receptor antagonist has recently been purified, sequenced, cloned, and expressed as a recombinant protein in *E. coli*. This inhibitor has been effective in various *in vitro* experiments but more recently has been shown to reduce the lethality of endotoxin-induced shock in rabbits, thus heralding a new approach to the treatment of septicaemia associated with Gram-negative bacterial infection.

A further approach has been to use specific antibodies against cytokines in the treatment of human disease. Natural antibodies to some cytokines, such as TNF-α and TNF-β are known to occur, but most research has focussed on the use of monoclonal antibodies, of either murine or human origin, since such antibodies can be developed relatively easily with hybridoma technology. Thus murine monoclonal antibodies to TNF have been shown to be effective in animal models of septic shock and trials in humans are currently taking place using such monoclonal antibodies. It will be of great interest to see whether specific cytokine antagonists are more effective than monoclonal antibodies against cytokines.

In conclusion, therapy with cytokines show great promise but numerous clinical trials involving large numbers of patients will be required to accurately define specific diseases and groups of patients who would benefit from cytokine therapy. Methods of reducing the toxicity associated with cytokine therapy are needed, since such toxicity is a serious obstacle to clinical advances in cytokine therapy. Nonetheless, cytokines are likely to be involved in major therapeutic advances in the next decade.

FURTHER READING

Arai, K., Lee, F., Miyajima, A., Miyatake, S., Arai, N. and Yokota, T. (1990) Cytokines: co-ordinators of immune and inflammatory responses. *Annual Reviews of Biochemistry*, **59**, 783–836.
Balkwill, F.R. and Burke, F. (1989) The cytokine network. *Immunology Today*, **10**, 299–304.
Meager, A. (1990) *Cytokines*. Open University Press, Milton Keynes.
Whitcher, J.T. and Evans, S.W. (1990) Cytokines in disease. *Clinical Chemistry*, **36**, 1269–1281.

Appendices

APPENDIX 1: PROTEIN STRUCTURES

Name	Size		Post-translational modifications				Plasma	Half-life
	kDa	Residues	CHO	Gla	Hydroxy	Sulphate	µg/ml	
Coagulation proteins								
Fibrinogen	340	3010	+	–	–	+	3000	4 d
A α	66*	625	–	–	–		–	–
B β	52*	469	+	–	–		–	–
γ	46*	411	+	–	–		–	–
Prothrombin	72	579	+	+	–	+	150	3 d
Factor V	286	2196	+	–	–		7	15 h
Tissue factor	45	263	+	–	–		0	–
Factor VII	50	406	+	+	–		0.5	4 h
Factor VIII	330	2332	+	–	–	+	0.3	18 h
von Willebrand factor	220*	2050	+	–	–		10	8 h
Factor IX	57	415	+	+	+		5	18 h
Factor X	59	445	+	+	+		10	2 d
Factor XI	80*	607	+	–			5	3 d
Factor XII	76	596	+	–			40	
Factor XIII	320						30	~10 d
A subunit	76*	731	–	–			20	–
B subunit	80*	641	+	–			10	–
Protein C	57	419	+	+	+	+	4	6 h
Protein S	69	635	+	+	+	+	29	42 h
Thrombomodulin	105	557	+	–			0	
Fibronectin	250*	2355	+	–		+	300	
Inhibitors								
Antithrombin-III	58	432	+	–	–	–	100	3 d
Heparin cofactor II	65	480	+	–	–	+	100	2.5 d
α₁-Protease inhibitor	52	394	+	–	–	–	1500	4 d
Antiplasmin	69	452	+	–	–	+	70	2.7 d
PAI-1	48	379	+				0.02	

PAI-2	60	415	+		0	
PAI-3/Protein C inhibitor	63	387	+		5	
Extrinsic path inhibitor	32	276	+	–	0.1	
α₂-Macroglobulin	185*	1451	+	–	2600	10.5 d
C₋₁-inhibitor	104	478	+	–	170	
Inter-α inhibitor	180*	–	+		10	
α H chain	92 to 107	≤544	+		–	
L chain	45	147	+		–	
Protease nexin 1	44	378	+		< 1	–
Fibrinolytic proteins						
Tissue-type plasminogen activator	65	527	+	–	0.05	3 min
Urokinase-type plasminogen activator	5	411	+	–	0.02	<10 min
Plasminogen	92	791	+	–	200	3 d
Histidine-rich glycoprotein	75	507	+	–	100	
Immunoglobulin						
IgG	150	~1300	+		12500	7 to 21 d
H chain	50*	~440	+		–	
L chain	25*	~220	+		–	
Albumin	68	585	–		40000	
Haemoglobin α/β	68 (17)*	141/146			(blood–10⁵)	
Cytokines						
IL-1	16	159/153	–			
IL-2	15	133	+		50 U/ml	
IL-3 (multi-CSF)	20 to 26	140/134	+			
IL-4	20	129	+			
IL-5	20	115	+			
IL-6 (IFN-β₂)	22 to 29	184				
Interferon-α/β	20 to 26	166/165	+			
Interferon-γ	143		+			
GM-CSF	22	127			0	–

(continued)

APPENDIX 1: PROTEIN STRUCTURES (continued)

Name	Size		Post-translational modifications				Plasma	Half-life
	kDa	Residues	CHO	Gla	Hydroxy	Sulphate	µg/ml	
G-CSF	20	174	+				<30pg/ml	–
M-CSF	47*	189 (522)	+				174U/ml	–
Erythropoietin	34	166	+				0.3ng/ml	8h
TNF-α	17	157	–				36U/ml	
TNF-β	25	171	+					
EGF	6	53						5min
TGF-α	13*	50 (160)						
TGF-β	25 (13)*	112 (390)						
PDGF-A/B	16/14*	≤124/109 (221/242)	±/–				0	2min
Basic FGF/HBGF-II	16	146						

* Protein composed of multiple subunits.

APPENDIX 2: GENE STRUCTURES

Name	Gene (kb)	Exons	mRNA (kb)	Chromosome	Year cDNA† cloned
Coagulation proteins					
Fibrinogen					
A α	50	5	2.2	4q 28–32	1984
B β	9	8	1.9		
γ	10	10	1.6		
Prothrombin	10.5	14	2.2	–	1983
Factor V	20.8	–	7		1987
Tissue factor	12.4	6	2.2 (3.2)	1p.ter	1987
Factor VII	12.8	9	~2	13q 3	1986
Factor VIII	186	26	9	Xq 28	1984
von Willebrand factor	178	52	9.5	12p 2	1985
Factor IX	34	8	2.8	Xq 26.27	1982
Factor X	22	8	1.4	13q 3	1985
Factor XI	23	15	2.1	–	1986
Factor XII	12	14	2.1	6p 23	1985
Factor XIII					
A subunit	–	–	3.8	6p 24	1986
B subunit	–	–	2.2	1q 31	1986
Protein C	11.6	8	1.8	2q 14.21	1984
Protein S	≤40	12	3.4	3pq	1986
Thrombomodulin	3.7	1	3.7	20	1987
Fibronectin	>40	>>10	complex	2q 32	1985
Inhibitors					
Antithrombin-III	19	7	1.5	1q 23.25	1983
Heparin Cofactor II	14.5	≥5	2.3	22	1987
α_1-Protease inhibitor	12.2	7	1.4 (1.8)	14q 31.32	1984
Antiplasmin	16	10	2.4	18p 11	1987
PAI-1	12.3	9	2.4 (3.4)	7q 21	1986
PAI-2	16.5	8	2.1 (1.5)	18q 21	1987
PAI-3/Protein C inhibitor	11.5	5	≥2.1	14	1987

(continued)

APPENDIX 2: GENE STRUCTURES (continued)

Extrinsic path inhibitor	–	–	1.4 (4.4)	–	1988
α₂-Macroglobulin	19	–	4.6	12	1985
C$_T$-Inhibitor		≥ 8	1.8	11p 11	1986
Inter-α inhibitor H/L	–/>4.6	–/>4	3.3/1.3	3p and 10/9q	1989/1988
Protease nexin 1		–	2.4	–	1988
Fibrinolytic proteins					
Tissue-type plasminogen activator	33	14	2.7	8p 12	1983
Urokinase-type plasminogen activator	6.4	11	2.4	10q 24	1985
Plasminogen	52.5	19	2.9	6q 25	1987
Histidine-rich glycoprotein	11	9	2.0	–	1986
Immunoglobulin					
IgG H chain	complex*	5	3	14	1978
L chain (K/L)	complex*	3	1.2	2/22	
Albumin	10	15	2.1	4q 11	1981
Haemoglobin α/β	0.8/1.6 (30/60)*	3/3	0.6/0.8	16p 12/11	1977
Cytokines					
IL-1	7.5	7	1.5	2q 13	1984
IL-2	4.5	4	1.1	4q 26	1983
IL-3 (multi-CSF)	2.3	5	1.3	5q 23.31	1986
IL-4	9	4	0.9	5q 23.31	1986
IL-5	3.2	4	1.1	5q 23.31	1987
IL-6 (IFN-β₂)	4.8	5	0.6	7p	1988
Interferon-α/β	1	1	1	9p 22	1980
Interferon-γ	5	4	1.5	12q 24	1982
GM-CSF	2.4	4		5q 23	1985
G-CSF	2.4	5	1.5	17q 21	1986
M-CSF	22	>11	1.8/4.8	5q 33	1985

Erythropoietin	5	5	1.4	7q 11	1984
TNF-α	2.7	4	1.8	6p 21	1984
TNF-β	2.0	4	1.6	6p 21	1984
EGF	110	24	5	4q 25	1985
TGF-α	–	–	4.8	2p 13	1984
TGF-β	4	7	2.5	19q 25	1985
PDGF: A/B	23/24	7/7	<2.8/3.5	7p/22q	1985
Basic FGF	≥34		2.2/4.6	4q	1986

* Gene cluster.

† Each year the journal *Nucleic Acids Research* lists, as an appendix, the known cloned protein genes with references.

APPENDIX 3A: SOME TYPES OF PLASMA-DERIVED PROTEIN CONCENTRATES

Factor VIII

Intermediate/high purity (<50U/mg)
8Y* (BPL)[1], Z8 (SNBTS), Profilate SD (α)[2], VIII:SD (NYBC)[2], Koate HS (Cutter)[2], Haemate P* (Behring)[3], etc.

Very high purity (>50 U/mg)
Octa VI (Octapharma)[2], VHP-VIII (Biotransfusion)[2], VIII-CP (Behring)[3], Koate-HP (Cutter)[3], etc.

Immunopurified (>1000 U/mg before albumin)
Monoclate P (Armour)[3], Hemofil M (Baxter)[2]

von Willebrand Factor

VHP-vWf (Biotransfusion)[2]

Factor IX

Prothrombin complex concentrate
(Prothrombin, FIX and FX with or without FVII: 9A (BPL)[1], DEFIX (SNBTS), Konyne (Cutter), Proplex (Baxter), Prothrombinex (CSL), PPSB (Biotransfusion)[2], Prothromplex (Immuno)[1], etc.

High-purity factor IX
VHP-IX (Biotransfusion)[2], Mononine (Armour), Alphanine (Alpha), Single FIX (Baxter/ARC)[2]

Activated prothrombin complex concentrates
FEIBA (Immuno)[1], Autoplex (Baxter), PAPC (Biotransfusion)

Factor VIII inhibitor therapeutics

Factors VII (BPL), Factor VII (Immuno), Acset (Biotransfusion)

Factor XI

Factor XI (BPL)

Factor XIII

Fibrogammin (Behring), Factor XIII (BPL)

Fibrin glue

Tisseel (Immuno)[1], Beriplast (Behring), Biocol (Biotransfusion)[2]

Thrombin

Human Thrombin (BPL; Dutch RC)
Bovine Thrombin (Behring; Immuno)

Antithrombin-III

Antithrombin-III (Kabi; BPL; Biotransfusion; Baxter; ARC; Immuno; Kofactor (Cutter)[3]

α₁-Protease inhibitor

Prolastin (Cutter)[3], Antitrypsin (Biotransfusion)

C-1-Inhibitor

C-1-Inactivator P (Behring)[3], C-₁-esterase inhibitor (Dutch RC)[3], C-1-esterase inhibitor (BPL)[3]

Immunoglobulin
Intramuscular
  Gammabulin (Immuno), Pentaglobin (Biotest)
Intravenous
  IVIgG (SNBTS), Sandoglobulin (Sandoz), Gammimmune N
  (Cutter), Gammagard (Baxter), Intraglobin (Biotest),
  Endobulin (Immuno)
Hyperimmune immunoglobulins
  Many – including concentrates of antibody to CMV,
  Vaccinia tetanus, Rhesus D, rabies, hepatitis B, varicella
  zoster, etc.

Albuminoids
Albumin[3]
Salt-poor protein solution ($\geq 85\%$ albumin)[3]

Notes
Steps taken to inactivate viruses include: (1) extended heat treatment of dried product; (2) use of solvent detergent; and (3) pasteurization.
* Also contains useful levels of vWf.

APPENDIX 3B: EXAMPLES OF SOME RECOMBINANT BLOOD-RELATED PRODUCTS AT CLINICAL TRIAL

Factor VIII (Recombinate, Baxter/Genetics Institute; Kogenate, Cutter/Genentech)

Factor VIIa (Niastase, Novo-Nordisk)

Tissue-type plasminogen activator (Actilyse, Genentech)

Urokinase-type plasminogen activator (pro UK; Sandoz, Genentech)

Erythropoietin (Eprox, Cilag Biotech; Recormon, Boehringer; Epogen, Amgen)

GM-CSF (Sandoz, Immunex, Schering Plough)

OKT3 murine monoclonal antibody (Ortho)

CAMPATH-1 monoclonal antibody (Wellcome)

Interferons (Amgen, Genentech, Biogen, Behringwerke, Cetus)

Tumour necrosis factor (BASF, Cetus, Genentech)

Interleukins, e.g. IL-2, IL-3

Hepatitis B surface antigen vaccine

APPENDIX 4: SUMMARY OF REQUIREMENTS FOR RECOMBINANT PARENTERAL THERAPEUTIC PRODUCTS

While each product is considered on its own merits, national and international author- ities have produced guidelines on possible general Regulatory requirements that should be met to assure the safety and efficacy of recombinant therapeutics. These are additional to those already required for conventional therapeutic products, e.g. tests for pyrogen and acute toxicity, although in some cases (*) a detailed knowledge of the native (plasma) product is required to undertake testing of the recombinant material.

The guideline proposals apply not only to recombinant therapeutics themselves, but also to any corresponding materials used to prepare them, such as monoclonal antibodies used in purification.

The suggested procedures are designed to test various aspects of safety and efficacy.

On cells used in the preparation of the product

- How to prepare and document master cell banks, working cell banks and prepare these from validated seed stock.
- Testing of these for any contamination by a range of bacteria viruses, mycoplasma or fungi (see below).
- Tests for genetic stability, tumourogenicity and identification (e.g. karyotyping or isoenzyme analysis).
- In the case of monoclonal antibodies, documentation of immunogen, immuniza- tion, animal stock and cellular fusion partner.
- For recombinant products, details of the genetic material (e.g. the recombinant plasmid) and manipulations used to prepare the master cell bank.

Tests on culture media

- To include tests for microorganisms (see below), endotoxin, etc.

Validation of the preparation process

- Demonstration of the batch-to-batch reproducibility of cell culture and subsequent product purification. This would include tests for genetic stability (see above).
- Demonstration of the stability of cell cultures over times greater than those used in production, be this by batch or continuous culture methods.
- Demonstration that the purification method removes potential viral contaminants, e.g. by model studies in which test virus is purposefully added (spiking studies).
- The usual guidelines on good manufacturing practice (Appendix 5) are applicable.

Tests on the product

- For contaminants, these could include:
  for viruses, e.g. by testing rodent production of anti-viral antibodies, tests for specific nucleic acids or reverse transcriptase (to detect retroviruses)
  for bacterial, mycoplasma, fungal or endotoxin contamination
  for cellular or viral nucleic acid (possible limit around <10 pg per dose) e.g. by hybridization, specific probing for oncogenic sequences or polymerase chain reaction to detect specific viral sequences

for residual cellular or media proteins (possible limit <10 µg per dose)
for any ligands (e.g. monoclonal antibody) leaked from materials used during
   purification
- To demonstrate identity, these could include:
assay of activity and specific activity*
amino acid composition*
tests of primary structure, e.g. peptide mapping and (partial) sequencing*
analysis of post-translational modifications, e.g. glycosylation, carboxylation,
   sulphation or hydroxylation*
physico-chemical properties, e.g. spectroscopy, chromatographic behaviour in at
   least two distinct systems, isoelectric focussing, electrophoresis in denaturing
   and non-denaturing systems, etc.
immunochemical analysis, e.g. reaction with appropriate, but not inappropriate,
   antibodies. This includes tests for neoantigens arising for non-native folding,
   aggregation, degradation or absence of normal modifications. Antibody
   products should be tested for reaction with the target antigen and a range of
   human tissues
- Other
possible testing for stability or efficacy (in animal models)
toxicology, mutagenicity and oncogenic testing in various animal species

---

* Detailed knowledge of the native (plasma) product required for testing of the recombinant
   material.
For further reading see listing after Appendix 5.

APPENDIX 5: GOOD MANUFACTURING PRACTICE (GMP) AND RELATED MATTERS

Manufacturers of pharmaceutical products are required, as one would expect, to meet certain quality standards. In the United States, inspection is carried out by the FDA (Food & Drugs Adminstration) and in the United Kingdom by the Medicines Inspectorate (MI). Similar systems exist elsewhere and operate on similar principles. In the United Kingdom, there is a requirement for manufacturers to obtain manufacturing and individual product licences. Inspections are carried out according to the principles set out in a booklet entitled *The Guide to Good Pharmaceutical Manufacturing*. This is more commonly known as *The Orange Guide*.

The guide defines three basic terms within the overall goal of ensuring that a product is of the appropriate quality for its intended use:

- *Quality assurance (QA)*
  Was originally intended to cover all aspects from initial process design to final storage of appropriately labelled product including GMP and QC. The term 'total quality management' (TQM) is coming into use and is intended to be of rather wider aspect, including such things as providing background information for staff and their motivation.
- *Good Manufacturing Practice (GMP)*
  Describes the process of documenting and recording all steps of production to ensure consistent manufacture of the product, and includes appropriate staff training and provision of premises.
- *Quality control*
  Is the sampling, specification and testing of not only the product, but also raw materials, packaging, etc.

Acceptable standards for setting up appropriate quality systems are defined in terms of:

- *Personnel and training*
  Production and quality control should be managed by clearly defined personnel (with appropriate deputies). Training of all staff should be according to written procedures and include an induction period, with periodic assessment of both staff and procedures.
- *Documentation*
  There is a great emphasis on this. It includes not only a specification of the product and detailed description of the process, but also of raw materials, packaging, intermediate products, distribution, storage and handling of any complaints. Guidelines are given on the layout, checking and review of documents, such as the record of each production batch. Descriptions of methods – standard operating procedures (SOPs) – should be unambiguous and easily followed. Such documentation is very helpful in developing QA structures.
- *Premises and equipment*
  These should be appropriate for the task and maintained in clean, working order, Guidance is given on items such as hygiene, appropriate air conditioning, specification of distinct storage areas, maintenance of records and servicing.
- *Manufacture*
  This should be carried out according to a declared, detailed written procedure using materials issued from a quarantined, validated stock. Any deviation from the procedure must be recorded, as should all materials used, the results of in-

process and final product sampling and of routine checks for contamination. All of this should be validated by regular audit.

- *Good control laboratory practice*
  Assessment of premises, equipment, cleanliness, reagents, sampling materials and their specification, together with the documentation of methods and recording of results should be performed by distinct personnel from those involved in production, although the latter should obviously be involved. While analysis may be subcontracted outwith the organization, the quality-control function cannot. Again, clear documentation and recording of the above should be established.
- *Other matters*
  Guidance is also given on appropriate approaches to the re-use of recovered materials and to establishing complaints and recall procedures. The latter include the establishment of investigation methods following recall of products associated with an adverse effect.

FURTHER READING

Cartwright, T. (1987) Isolation and purification of products from animal cells. *Trends in Biotechnology*, **5**, 25–30.

Committee for Proprietary Medicinal Products (1989) Notes to Applicants for Marketing Authorisations on the Pre-clinical Biological Safety Testing of Medicinal Products Derived from Biotechnology. *Journal of Biological Standardization*, **17**, 203–212.*

Committee for Proprietary Medicinal Products (1989) Notes to Applicants for Marketing Authorisation on the Production and Quality Control of Monoclonal Antibodies of Murine Origin Intended for Use in Man. *Journal of Biological Standardization*, **17**, 213–222.

Committee for Proprietary Medicinal Products (1989) Notes to Applicants for Marketing Authorisation on the Production and Quality Control of Medicinal Products Derived by Recombinant DNA Technology. *Journal of Biological Standardization*, **17**, 223–231.*

FDA (1987) Points to Consider in the Manufacturing and Testing of Monoclonal Antibody Products for Human Use. Report issued by the U.S. Food & Drugs Administration, Office of Biologics.

FDA (1985) Points to Consider in the Production and Testing of New Drugs and Biologics Produced by Recombinant DNA Technology. Report issued by the U.S. Food & Drugs Administration.

Medicines Inspectorate. *The Guide to Good Pharmaceutical Manufacturing*, HMSO. Prepared by the Medicines Inspectorate of the Departments of Health and Social Security.

Sauer, F. (1989) EEC Guidelines on Medicinal Products Derived from Modern Biotechnology Process. *Journal of Biological Standardization*, **17**, 201–202.

* Summarized in a supplement in *Trends in Biotechnology*, 7 February 1989.

Index

Index compiled by Caroline Sheard